# THE PHYSICIAN'S GUIDE TO THE BUSINESS OF MEDICINE: DREAMS AND REALITIES

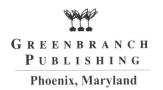

GREENBRANCH
PUBLISHING

Phoenix, Maryland

## JEFFREY T. GORKE

Copyright © 2010 by Greenbranch Publishing, LLC
ISBN: 978-0-9814738-0-2

Published by Greenbranch Publishing, LLC
PO Box 208
Phoenix, MD 21131
Phone: (800) 933-3711
Fax: (410) 329-1510
Email: info@greenbranch.com
Website: www.mpmnetwork.com, www.soundpractice.net, www.codapedia.com

This publication is designed to provide general medical practice management information and is sold with the understanding that neither the author nor the publisher is engaged in rendering legal, accounting, ethical, or clinical advice. If legal or other expert advice is required, the services of a competent professional person should be sought.

CPT® is a registered trademark of the American Medical Association.

Printed in the United States of America by United Book Press, Inc. www.unitedbookpress.com

PUBLISHER
Nancy Collins

EDITORIAL ASSISTANT
Jennifer Weiss

BOOK DESIGNERS
Laura Carter
Stephanie Rohde

INDEX
Paul Hightower

COPYEDITOR
Sarah Herndon

# PRAISE FOR JEFF GORKE

"After completing medical school and residency, physicians are well trained to take care of patients, but have had virtually no guidance or experience with the practice of medicine within the complicated and chaotic American health care system. While they may know everything about diagnosing and treating their patients, young physicians often enter medical practice with little or no understanding of the complexities of the business aspects of health care. When they first enter practice, most physicians have no concept of how to work within and manage their medical practice, which, in most cases, is a small corporation or business. From negotiating with insurance companies to managing an office staff to working with other physicians who are now their business partners, most young physicians enter practice with little idea of what they're getting themselves into. Jeff Gorke's book is an excellent introduction to this complicated world. In an informal and straight-forward manner, Gorke first advises young physicians on how to find a job and negotiate an employment contract. He then explains the nuts and bolts of the business of medical practice, including administrative structure and functioning, how medical care is reimbursed, and basic practice finance. The book is an excellent primer for any physician about to enter medical practice."

MICAH R. TEPPER, MD, FACC
*Atlanta, GA*


"This book is a must read for every physician preparing to enter the complex world of private practice, regardless of the setting. Book One superbly presents every one of the major and minor decision points that should be considered before these physicians embark on their quest to find the 'right' practice. Clearly explained, in great detail, is the multitude of procedures to follow from the preparation of one's CV to the process for the employment agreement, once the 'right' practice has been found (and all of the steps in between). Book Two, dealing with "the nuts and bolts of a private practice," should be read by these same physicians and also by their many colleagues who, although in private practice for years, are still overwhelmed by the complexities and intricacies of the business of healthcare."

JULIA C. LEWIS, RN, MS
*Practice Management Consultant*
*Lady Lake, FL*

"Finally, there comes a book that prepares the freshly minted physician for the business side of the healthcare equation. Mr. Gorke's light, easy-to-digest style takes the reader, from soup to nuts, through the entire process of determining and finding the right practice setting; and then, in the same fashion, through the myriad of real-life business, governance, and management issues that every physician will face. Not only is this for physicians, it should be part of all residency programs."

KENNETH J. LOPEZ
*Radiology Administrator*
*Longview, WA*


"Jeff has written a great instructional tool for any MD who is either new to the business of medicine and looking to relocate, or is currently in residency contemplating the interviewing phase of his or her life. Jeff has laid out a practical, logical, and systematic approach to help any physician identify, quantify, and evaluate potential new employers and future business partners. The illustrations, charts, and anecdotal information are easy to understand, shed light on traditionally difficult information, and keep the reader focused all the way through. The book should be required reading for physicians to assist them in their career search and to clarify and explain in a practical way the 'business' of medicine."

WILLIAM (BILL) L. HUGHES, CPA, CMPE
*Administrator*
*Women's Health Specialists*
*Jensen Beach, FL*

# DEDICATION

*For her endless optimism, an abiding belief, and the strength
of the ages, I humbly dedicate this book to my best friend and
dear wife, Pam. She is the bond to reality, the keeper of the flame,
and the champion of the underdog. Pam, I love you.*

# ACKNOWLEDGMENTS

AS THE SAYING GOES, NO MAN IS AN ISLAND. No statement more accurately reflects that sentiment than the work you are about to read. I'm indebted to friends and associates in the expansive community that is the United States health care system who've offered creative thoughts, ideas, and input to assure that this book is as comprehensive and thorough as possible, given its design and premise.

Many individuals contributed their valuable time to vetting this effort. I'm truly grateful. Yet I take full responsibility for any missteps or foibles contained herein.

# TABLE OF CONTENTS

## BOOK ONE: The Job Search

*And so it begins*

## BOOK TWO: On to Business

*The nuts and bolts of the private practice*

# ABOUT THE AUTHOR

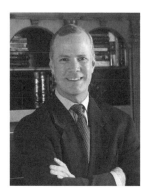 Jeff Gorke has been involved in the craziness of health care and health care management for 20 years. He is the President and Chief Executive Officer of Castle Gate Management (www.castlegatemanagement.com), a health care management advisory and health care information technology company. His experience ranges from Medicare administration to running both large and small, single-specialty, privately-held medical group practices to medical society management on a national level.

Jeff holds a Bachelor of Business Administration from Temple University in Philadelphia, with majors in both finance and international business, and a Masters of Business Administration from the University of Richmond in Richmond, Virginia.

Jeff, his wife Pam, and their daughters live outside of Atlanta, Georgia.

For more information, please contact Jeff Gorke at Castle Gate Management, info@castlegatemanagement.com or (888) 439-2558.

# FOREWORD

SEARCHING FOR A JOB AS A PHYSICIAN is a daunting task given how poorly medical school prepares one for it. There are many factors to consider as you begin this process, and Jeff Gorke does a wonderful job simplifying this complex topic. We doctors have trained for years learning medicine, so it's not surprising how little we know about the business side of our chosen career. With 20 years of experience in managing medical practices, Jeff is able to simplify what may be one of the most important choices you will ever make.

After finishing my fellowship, I joined a large single-specialty cardiology practice in Florida. My eyes widened in awe as I walked into the four-story main office building. The ground floor had a beautiful cath lab with multiple recovery rooms, each with its own TV. Other floors housed the research department, administration, and patient care areas. I couldn't wait to sign the contract and be a part of this magnificent practice! If only I had read this book, my first my thoughts would have been a little more realistic: How much overhead does all this represent, how hard are the partners working to support this building, who owns this property, and, of course, what kind of compensation are the doctors receiving? Not surprisingly, I rushed to sign the contract thinking I might lose the job to some other physician. It was an almost fatal error that cost me two years of my life and nearly ruined my marriage.

The fancy overhead was indeed a major problem for this group as we worked extremely hard with incomes far below the national average. The practice was generally run by a handful of original partners who controlled most aspects of the business. When a partner suddenly quit, a cascade of mistrust ensued, eventually leading to the break-up of this 30-year-old practice. It was a good practice, an honest practice but one that could not survive its overhead, leadership structure, and internal mistrust. I vowed to learn about the business side of medicine so this would never happen again to my family and me. And so far, it hasn't!

I spent six months looking for a new life, my path closely following the many topics Jeff reviews in this book. I learned that the type of practice is as important as its location (small practice, larger group, hospital employed, etc.). I decided upon a medium-sized private group that would be large enough to have multiple revenue streams, be able to negotiate with private insurance companies, enjoy cheaper malpractice costs, and have a better retirement plan.

The culture of a group is also critically important. Know what your values are, and find a group that shares them. Our group values cost-effective, evidence-based care and a quality lifestyle for its physicians and employees. A doctor primarily focused on income would be miserable in my group. Know yourself and know your group. Jeff explains that finding the practice of your choice is only the first part of this process. You need to understand the inner workings of the group such as its governance structure, buy-in, buy-out, compensation model, practice reputation, local competition, and physician internal dynamics. This all sounds like a daunting task, and without the help of this book, it would be. I interviewed with all the members of my practice paying special attention to the senior partners. From there, I spoke to the nurses in the hospitals, cath lab techs, and MDs who had left the practice. Do your homework first before you sign the contract.

No matter which type of practice you enter, the external pressures on medicine are forcing each and every one of us to become businesspeople. Like it or not, you have to learn these basic skills or you will be walked over by the hospitals, the government, and possibly even your partners. I'm not suggesting you panic or become disillusioned, it's just a fact of modern-day practice. Jeff does a wonderful job of explaining how physicians are compensated by various entities, the use of RVUs, and proper coding with documentation. Once you gain this knowledge and skill set, you can finally focus on the enjoyment of the practice of medicine. I can honestly tell you I love practicing medicine and have come to find the business side equally as interesting.

This book is the tool you need to develop both your medical and business careers. Jeff's guidance has helped me immensely through the years, and I owe him a debt of gratitude. You will too.

STEVEN J. ISSERMAN, MD, FACC
*Director of Echo Lab, Sleep/DME Program, and Clinical Research*
*Western Piedmont Heart Centers*
*Conover, NC*

# PREAMBLE

CONGRATULATIONS ON THE PURCHASE OF THIS BOOK. I'd like to think that you've made an exceedingly wise buying decision—no, a wise investment decision—with this acquisition. It's my hope that this book will serve as a mini-MBA of sorts for you. If it does, it will save you from the wear and tear of more schooling and will offer you tidbits of what is needed to be functional on the business side of the field you've chosen. There are a smattering of joint MD/MBA programs available to physicians today, but frankly, I'm not quite sure that you need a full-blown MBA to get accomplished what you need to when you enter private practice. Why would I suggest such a thing? First, many of you may not use 90% or more of the MBA education you'd accumulate, rendering about all but a couple months of a two-year program, well, a waste of your time. Second, why go through the cost and expense when you can read this fine tome and gain at least a basic understanding, possibly all you'll need, to move yourself forward in the "business" of medicine?

The time required to read and digest the contents herein should prove a good investment in your continuing education vis-à-vis the private practice of health care. At least from my perspective.

The goals of this book are broad but fairly simple:

1.  to assist new physicians down a logical path toward a good employment decision (vs. a bad train wreck),
2.  to offer any/all MDs a basic look at the "business" of medicine in an attempt to place them higher on the learning curve re: same,
3.  to offer insight into what's inside the private practice, and,
4.  to entertain with some anecdotes gleaned during nearly 20 years in this sometimes crazy business. (Author's note: the examples provided are from third party recountings. They are real. The names have been changed to protect the innocent. Of course they're true: who could make this stuff up!?)

The aforementioned goals are wide-reaching, lofty, and entail a great bit of depth and detail. The problem with a book as general as this is that you cannot hit, in absolute, all things as they pertain to all specialties or all variations within the complicated health care animal. That being the case, I've tried to paint, in wide strokes and with a big brush, what an MD might expect as s/he looks toward employment. Though much of this can be summed in fairly general terms, I don't wish to oversimplify the business of medicine. Many of the topics I've peripherally dipped my toes into in this book have had full texts constructed about them. I considered that a more generic, flyover look would offer you a better understanding than many of your predecessors had. And if I get this non-exhaustive laundry list accomplished, even in minor measure, you should have culled a valuable nugget or two out of this exercise.

Keep in mind that, although this book speaks to many things germane to the business side of the practice of medicine, it is decidedly geared toward the practitioner who seeks employment in a private practice setting. After all, that is where a majority of you will end up.

I've tried to keep this book somewhat light. By that I mean plenty of detail without the parched, tasteless delivery of a textbook. This book was written to be aerodynamic and designed for speed, because your time, like all of ours, is precious. And your time will become even more precious to you. Your "own" time is soon, once you get into practice, to devolve into a few stolen moments while you commute to/from work. So I've written this with as much detail as I could in a manner that'll enable you to read it quickly. Where possible and practical, I've employed spreadsheets and graphical depictions because I'm a visual kind of guy. And as they say, a picture's worth a thousand words. You can throw contracts and assorted legal mumbo-jumbo at me, but if I can't see those words boiled down into hard figures, I'm about lost. Besides, seeing some numbers in action will be of practical value to you.

## Genesis

The genesis of this book was quite simple. In interviewing a handful of physicians during 2005, I was struck by what these highly educated folks did not know about what they were about to embark upon. Considered this way, you are about to step into a sword fight against three competitors and you have no sword and are blindfolded. That should be an apt analogy.

Many of these new MDs did not know how they, or their practices, were paid by the various entities that, for all intents and purposes, set their prices. They were unsure of what overhead truly was. They didn't know what to look for in terms of managers, consultants, or business structure. To make matters worse, they were sure of neither the business side of the practice nor the shareholder ("partner") side. All, by and large, new ideas for the young Fellow, or even the physician who's been practicing for a couple of years but has been outside of the running of the business.

I realized that in this niche, if I could offer a primer of sorts, even for MDs with some experience in the trenches, I would offer a valuable service. See, most MDs don't have time to go hither and yon to learn about practice management and the job search process. If they have dedicated CME time available, more than likely they'll use it to get better at what they do, which is to deliver high quality medicine. But physicians have a need, an urgent need, to understand the business side of medicine. The problem is that the actual practice of medicine seems to keep most MDs busy; go figure.

The day-to-day of practice management is time-consuming and laborious. Even if you had the time, you might not be able to keep up. As long as I've been in this business I still find myself running ragged. But as the soon-to-be owner of a medical practice and small business, it's essential that you at least understand the nuts and bolts of the thing. You don't need to be overly involved day-to-day, you just need to know.

## *Further Thoughts*

If you learn one thing about me in reading this book, I hope you'll learn that I'm a quality guy. For me, there's a duality to the phrase "quality guy." To wit, I like to think I'm a good, upstanding, thoughtful, and considerate guy, but I also mean, in the parameters of this book, that I'm pro-clinical quality and efficient delivery of care. That's the type of quality I'm referring to. And I'm a stickler for it and a big fan of it.

A private medical practice is a business. It operates along the razor-fine margin between the application of business methods and models and the art and science of medicine. But it is a business, make no mistake about it. As such, in your time you'll probably borrow money (as a corporation), have clinical quality measures and measurements, have accounting checks and balances, have collections practices to assure money is flowing into the practice, finance a profit-sharing plan, and probably pay taxes. As you enter into the labyrinth that is practice management and private practice, you may just find you know a lot less than you think.

This book is not meant to be an absolute in terms of a roadmap to medical practice success and it offers no guarantees. The intent is not to oversimplify a series of very complex systems. Also, I don't offer legal or financial advice. Instead, my goal is to offer new physicians and other clinicians a basic understanding of what they'll face in the private practice environment, from a fairly high level.

This book is the product of many years in this industry and bearing witness to a fair amount of changes. After my physician-interviewing epiphany, I got to thinking that maybe, just maybe, there was a market for this type of "MD self-help book," if you will. I think you'll agree and hope you find this to be a resource in your arsenal.

I've tried to build this book in terms of its flow of material, the logical—as I view it—management of content with regard to how your job search process will evolve, and what to look for when you've identified a practice. This book is decidedly a didactic tool to help you understand the practical side of pondering a clinical career, obtaining the position of interest, and happily "living" with that decision. One thing I hate to hear about is clinicians who stumble into a job they think is "the one" only to learn about nuances, caveats, and "we'll take care of yous" once they have arrived and started to practice. They've probably been set up, with no willful or wanton intent, to fail. The job search is not as covert a process in those terms as it is overt, but many physicians "fail" (not defined as clinical failure but failure to fit) because of what they don't know going into a job.

In any event, this book should serve as a tool and guide. It is chock-full of material designed to get you examining the next step(s) in your work-life with a different, more critical and objective eye.

What I endeavor to do is offer you what you missed in your medical training: a practical look at a medical practice. What I hope this does for you is allow you to make a good, comprehensive decision about which practice you choose and the direction your professional life will take. The more you control going in, the more fulfilled and satisfied you'll be. You'll find that making many of these decisions up front will allow you to enter your next phase of life "eyes open." The fewer surprises, the better off all of you will be.

From time to time, you'll find me using trite and tired business vernacular. But like it or not, some time ago medicine crossed into the realm of business. Philosophically, though it may be distasteful to the gentle reader, the two need not be mutually exclusive. If you don't buy into that philosophy, you may want to remain in academics.

Once again, and with authority, this book is no magic bullet, no key to success, no elixir served from a holy chalice. It is one of many tools you will use in learning about the business side of medicine that will impact you from your first day in the private practice of medicine.

And, you may or may not know, Current Procedural Terminology codes (CPT®) are the sole product of the American Medical Association (AMA) and are used with grateful attribution to the AMA. All rights reserved by AMA.

One last takeaway: I'm no attorney. The thoughts, musings, and ramblings I render herewith should neither be construed as legal, accounting, nor professional advice.

And so, on to the nuts and bolts. Good luck. Call if you need some help.

# BOOK ONE

# The Job Search

## AND SO IT BEGINS

### First Things First

YOU ARE A PHYSICIAN. You should have no problem getting a job. There is a very real need for more physicians and as the population in the US ages, the need for more physicians will continue unabated. Patient encounters per physician will continue to grow, the workload will increase, and certain stressors may leach into your life.

That said, this book does not contemplate whether or not you'll get a job. Presupposing that you will find a job, this book offers insight into what to look for when hunting down that new job or transitioning from one practice to the next. It strives to help you understand the business of medicine.

### Introspection

In a perfect world, and done properly, your career search would be a well thought-out and duly contemplated endeavor. Many of the topics and approaches I suggest are those that you may ponder or follow through with subconsciously vs overtly performing. I believe that putting some structure to your job search process better enables you to analyze and weigh the data relevant to your search and, in the end, it goes a long way to providing you overall satisfaction with your job choice.

### The Pyramid

I'm going to build you a very fundamental and simple pyramid. It'll offer you a graphic representation of how your search process might progress. A pyramid, of course, is the type of structure that incorporates a broad and stable base, essentially the foundation, which leads to the stacking of other "bricks" or levels culminating at an endpoint, the top. Those building blocks are metaphors for the segments in your job search process that meld to build a structured avenue to landing a position that you will enjoy. The "nifty graphic" below was unapologetically pulled from the US Department of Agriculture's new and improved "food pyramid." Picture yourself as the little food pyramid climber, climbing your way to career nirvana.

As you probably already know, where *you* want to be is integral to career fulfillment and ultimate satisfaction with life. You spend, minimally, 8 hours a day, 40 hours a week, at your job. You will usually spend more waking hours at work than at home. That said, you had better love what you do and where you do it or you've already set yourself up for disaster and emotional pain.

Your off-the-job happiness is just as important as your on-the-job happiness. And if you're married, or have a significant other who may be accompanying you on your next stage in life, finding co-nirvana in whatever location you identify is essential. Perhaps you are a Fellow with 6–9 months left in training or you're a physician in a setting that's not quite what you'd expected (because you didn't have access to this book) and you're looking to make a change. You're in a transitional period of your life and I'm hoping to help you move on to the next level armed with some knowledge that will impact your decision.

The lynchpin as you begin your search is a considerable level of internal honesty and introspection divining where you want to spend the next 5 to 10 to 20 years practicing medicine. Do you want to practice near family or as far away from family as is humanly possible without leaving the comfort of the continental 48 states? Do you love the coast (left or right)? If you're married, well, you know your spouse is going to have some input into that equation if you want to maintain matrimonial harmony and marital bliss. Where does s/he want to be? These questions should serve as the foundation, the building blocks, to crafting a decision pyramid that will point you to the perfect practice.

## DECISION PYRAMID — FOUNDATION

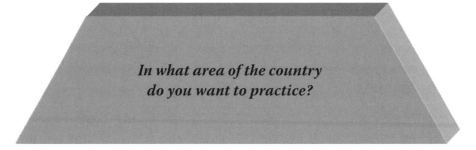

*In what area of the country
do you want to practice?*

Criteria for "Where"
- Lifestyle choices and inputs (in no particular order)

- Dining, arts & leisure, sports, area traffic/mass transportation
- Religious worship
- School systems
- Practice opportunity
  - Area opportunities in your specialty and setting

Laying the foundation of the pyramid, we'll begin by analyzing where in the country you want to be. We'll then consider the type of practice you wish to be a part of. Once you've conquered these components, you've handled a fair piece of the overall puzzle. At that point, you can winnow your hunt down to more specific regions, local areas, and groups. Generally speaking, the salient components in your job search, and thus the building blocks of the pyramid, boil down to a handful of key points:

1. In the geographic area of interest to you, what is the physician penetration? How many MDs are there per 100,000 people?
   a. More specifically, how many physicians are there in *your specialty* per 100,000 people?

2. What type of group or practice setting do you want to be in? Academic, hospital-based, private practice, multi-specialty group? Will your choice limit *where* you can practice? That is, academic opportunities in your specialty may not be offered in the area of the country in which you want to be.

3. What is the patient demographic? Does your chosen geographic area have an older or younger population? Is the crux of the patient mix "healthier" or "sicker?" For instance, in the greater Washington, DC area there might be less demand for cardiologists per capita than there is, say, in Anywhere, Mississippi (Mississippi being one of the "fattest" states according to *Trust for America's Health*[1]) which may mean that in DC they may "use" less cardiovascular health care per patient for a large city.

4. What is the payer "mix" in the area? Does Medicare (a notoriously poor payer that pays timely) dominate?
   a. Would Medicare be a dominant payer in your specialty in your area of choice? For instance, ophthalmic surgery in Florida. Or are the "Blues" the biggest payer?

5. What is the med/mal overview for the area? Are MDs in that area being haunted by med/mal scenarios that are out of control? Are juries "left" or "right" leaning in how they approach med/mal cases? And, is your specialty a target? Med/mal insurers take into consideration specialty trends as a component in pricing their med/mal rates. They also evaluate the area to determine if it's a sue-happy environment.

# I.  MD Market Saturation

The numbers of physicians, and even physician extenders, in a given area can impact the quality of your practicing life, which can impact the quality of your personal life. When evaluating a practice, if the ideal location is an ideal location for other MDs (eg, a large metropolitan area, good quality of life, etc), then you can expect to have more physicians vying more competitively for the available patient base, which may ultimately lower compensation. Why would that be? At first, I was going to opine that it's less supply/demand driven, in a classical sense. Yet it really is a matter of simple economics, when you boil it down. There is demand by physicians who want to be in a metro area with a corresponding limited supply of jobs in that area for that specialty. And the market will ultimately determine the going rate of pay in that area vs other areas in the country where the supply in a given specialty is low and the corresponding compensation is a bit higher. I know of a quasi-metro area in the country where a specialist was offered $180,000 to join a group and start practicing right out of Fellowship. The cost of living was fairly high. Yet in a southern state, I've seen that same position go for more than $225,000, even though the southern state in question had a significantly lower cost of living.

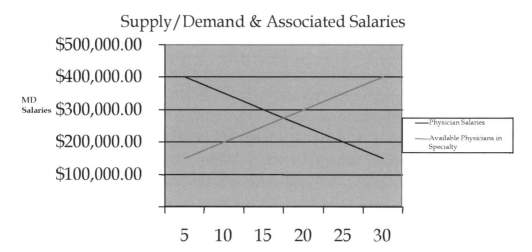

Though the example above is oversimplified, you get the picture (literally). If there are less bodies to fill available jobs, as indicated by the lighter line that rises as it moves from left to right (indicating about 5 MDs at the low end and about 30 at the high end), then there should be higher compensation as you must pay more to drive more physicians into the area (eg, the dark line starting high at approximately $400,000 and dropping to approximately $150,000 on the low end). In large metro areas, there are usually a significant number of physicians for slots available, thereby increasing demand for jobs and driving down compensation plans. In the graph above, on the y-axis, you see a fictional representation of physician salaries and on the x-axis you note the number of physicians in a specialty in a geographic area. As you might surmise, as the number of available physicians in a given area in a given specialty *increases* (again, the lighter line that increases from approximately 5 physicians), the corresponding amount of pay the market will bear begins to decline. From the graph above you can see that there is a certain market equilibrium achieved in this specialty and marketplace for about 17 physicians at $275,000 per year (where the light and dark lines intersect). As more MDs arrive in the market, the number on the x-axis increases (light line), and the compensation line (dark line) moves south as it moves from left to right and compensation decreases.

Let's look at this in real terms. If you're a radiologist and you want to be in New York City, you might reasonably expect that there are a bazillion other radiologists who'd like to flock to the bright lights and big city for the quality of life, shopping, and cultural aesthetic. That said, that desire to be in a big metro area means that the established groups in that area can pick and choose who they hire, knowing that the supply should be good. Market forces really determine who will be added and at what cost.

Aside from the supply/demand of MDs relative to compensation, more MDs in a market can translate directly into more marketing costs. How? Well, if you're in a highly competitive market, you'll need to make sure your name is out there to attract patients and to establish yourself, whether you're a solo practitioner or joining a larger group. Certainly, there are efficiencies to be gained in terms of marketing dollars when you join a well-seasoned group with a good name in the community. But you must contemplate marketing akin to separating the wheat from the chaff. Remember, your best, read that again, your **best** and least costly form of marketing is word of mouth. And make sure that you have good relationships with referring clinicians and offer the best quality of care and responsiveness available.

As a new physician in a new area, you might expect to have to spend a little cash (or the practice will) to assure that referring physicians or the general public know your name. As an aside, just so you know, your marketing cash cannot go into the pockets of referring physicians. That's a definite no-no, what they call a potential *inducement to refer*. But if there are multiple MDs battling for limited patient "eyes," this might mean added cost in terms of marketing (as you'll be advertising your "business") so that you can draw more patients to your group than your competition draws. In less competitive areas, there exists little if any need to "work" for patients (defined for our purposes as marketing), since patients will be available for you. In a highly competitive area, you'll need to differentiate yourself from your competition.

## II. Patient Demographics

Intuitively, there exist areas in the country that require less care for patient segments than others. Certainly, the demand for ophthalmologists might be higher in Florida where there exists a larger senior patient population who might require cataract surgery.

Understanding where the patients are relative to where you want to be is important, and dovetails with your consideration vis-à-vis physician saturation and practice type. There also exist areas where patients are more sophisticated relative to their health care. That is, some patients are more informed and take a vested and more active interest in their health care and some, frankly, do not. This may come into play in how you deliver care.

## III. Payer Mix

Payer mix is of interest to a clinician changing jobs or a new clinician, as it correlates to how much effort is required to pay the bills and have a little left over to pay the physicians. For instance, in areas of the country where managed care, in its purer sense of the phrase, is still formidable, (by that I mean capitated, or cap, plans), how you are paid is dependant upon on the patient population and a "per member per month" (pmpm) calculation. Per member, per month, in its broadest sense, means you receive a capitated amount of money (capped off) for each member in the plan for each month. Let us say that Highway Robbery Plan has 100 patients in California and they pay your practice $50 pmpm each month. You know that you'd generate $5,000 each month from the plan ($50 pmpm × 100 patients). Should that contract run for one year, you would be compensated $60,000 (12 months × $5,000/month) for treating those patients. Here, as you might imagine, is the rub. That $60,000 *might* be ok as long as it didn't cost you $70,000 to treat that patient population. And that is where the cap plans get a little murky. If you can treat those patients efficiently and spend only, say, $55,000 treating them, you'd earn $5,000 from that plan. This is an *at risk* contract. Why? Because you are *at risk* for spending more to treat the patient than you might receive in compensation for the care given. To add another fly in the ointment, the number of patient visits is **not** capped. In other words, patients can see you as often as either you, or they, feel is necessary.

You can see how the calculus for this plan works. There is a considerable amount *at risk*, meaning you are unsure what it will end up costing you to treat that patient population. Admittedly, I don't deal with these plans too frequently and they have diminished in size and scope over the last 10–20 years. Much of the pmpm game has been a West coast phenomenon. But these cap plans can pose very real management questions to be answered. Your skilled practice administrator will need to know the possible cost to care for treating the patient population of Highway Robbery Plan, how sick they are, and what might be required in terms of treatment protocols. S/he must then know acutely the cost to run your practice, and the opportunity cost of being "in network" for other plans vs being in network for Highway Robbery. Remember, when you're seeing these Highway Robbery patients, there are other patients, maybe on better reimbursing plans, that you will not be seeing. This is a consideration and a component of this odd business where the practice of medicine butts up against the business of medicine.

## JEFF'S NON-EXHAUSTIVE MANAGED CARE CONTINUUM

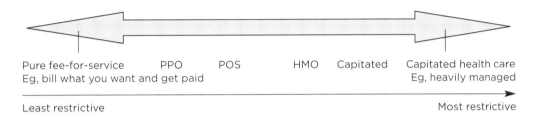

| Pure fee-for-service | PPO | POS | HMO | Capitated | Capitated health care |
| Eg, bill what you want and get paid | | | | | Eg, heavily managed |

Least restrictive → Most restrictive

***PPO (Preferred Provider Organization)*** = patient "self directs" or chooses his own physician in network. Provider offers care at "discounted fee" to members.[2]

***POS (Point of Service)*** = an option that allows members to choose to receive a service from a participating or non-participating clinician. Usually covered is reduced for use of an "out of network" provider.[3]

***HMO (Health Maintenance Organization)*** = an entity that provides, offers, or arranges coverage for designated health services for members for a fixed prepaid premium.[4]

***Capitated plan*** = dollar amount established to cover the cost of care for a member for a given period of time.[5]

In areas where a fair number of the plans are fee-for-service, your opportunities are better and your participation decisions less complex. Normally, you'll have a plan from Freeway Robbery Insurance (FRI), a subsidiary of Bleed 'Em Dry, Inc, where you have a contracted fee amount. Your charges in your group might be $100 for an office visit and FRI may agree to pay you $80 for that visit. So you know that each time you see Patient X, you'll receive $80. This won't hit against any cap or total amount that you can spend on Patient X's care. If you see Patient X 3 times during the month and perform nothing but office visits on him (where clinically appropriate), you know you'll receive $240 ($80 allowable × 3 visits). As you can see, were Patient X in Highway Robbery's capitated plan, you would have lost $190 on him. (pmpm for Highway Robbery = $50/month/pmpm; Patient X's actual 3 visits are $240 on FRI's fee-for-service plan. $50/pmpm – $240 = <$190>). Of course, this oversimplifies things a bit.

Yet what we've shown is there is an opportunity cost, a missed opportunity, of having Patient X as a member of a capitated plan vs having him on Freeway Robbery's fee-for-service plan. You might not have truly lost $190. The true loss is predicated on how much it actually costs you to render treatment to Patient X. But as you can see, there is a disparity for Patient X as a fee-for-service patient vs a capitated patient.

In areas of the country where Medicare is your largest payer, they may also be your worst payer in terms of revenue per procedure. Medicare is pretty darned good, pretty consistent, about paying on time. However, what they pay you is a different story. Medicare may pay you $100 for an office visit where Private Plan X might pay you $140. Wouldn't it be more financially beneficial to you if you saw a Private Plan X patient in your office instead of a Medicare patient? Yet some areas of the country are dominated by Medicare and Medicare Advantage Plans (or Medicare C plans): plans farmed out to third parties to administer. And the incessant drumbeat from our friends on Capitol Hill does not bode well for future reimbursement for the Medicare program. With each year, more and more cuts are on the way. As I write this book, there are rumblings about a 21% cut for 2010. Invariably, and historically, there has come a compromise in the 11th hour where the cuts are . . . well . . . cut. In 2008, the across-the-board planned cut was winnowed back. But the cut was still a cut and the cost to practice medicine did not get cut in kind.

In any event, given the scenario above, between Medicare and Private Plan X, more patient visits are required of the Medicare population to generate equivalent revenue for the business. Mind you, this does **not** mean less quality of care or scheduling unnecessary visits. It simply means the clinician must see more patients in a day to generate equivalent revenues.

**EXHIBIT 1.**

| I. | MEDICARE PAYMENTS | | PRIVATE PLAN X PAYMENTS | |
|---|---|---|---|---|
| | 10 | Patients | 10 | Patients |
| | $100 | Revenue per OV | $140 | Revenue per OV |
| | $1,000 | Total revenue | $1,400 | Total revenue |

To equate Medicare revenue to Private Plan X revenue, a clinician must see 4 more Medicare patients.

| II. | MEDICARE PAYMENTS | | PRIVATE PLAN X PAYMENTS | |
|---|---|---|---|---|
| | 14 | Patients | 10 | Patients |
| | $100 | Revenue per OV | $140 | Revenue per OV |
| | $1,400 | Total revenue | $1,400 | Total revenue |

What managed care means to many folks is the managing of care usually by deploying a gatekeeper approach. The gatekeeper might be an internal med doc or family practice doc who examines the patients and then refers them out to a specialist to treat whatever the ailing bodily system might be. The theory behind this is to control unnecessary visits to specialists by limiting access via the gatekeeper, who decides whether or not the patient needs to see a specialist. If not, the primary can treat and the insurance plan does not incur the cost of an unnecessary specialist visit and/or diagnostic test. Given the history of managed care and health care in general, this model has not faired too well in controlling health care costs.

As you can see, the insurance payer mix is an important component for a medical practice and clinician.

# IV. Med/Mal Overview

The medical malpractice component is an interesting one. Some areas of the country, and some specialties, have higher rates based on a multitude of factors. (It's sort of like the drug cost/price issue; is all the drug money in research or marketing?) But some med/mal carriers target higher risk specialties in higher risk markets to receive higher rates.

The type of specialty and risk involved will be one determinant to what you pay in med/mal. Are you performing complex cardiovascular surgery? If so, are you in a market where there have been multitudes of lawsuits brought by disgruntled patients? When pricing their products, med/mal carriers examine the socioeconomic demographic, the swing of the jury trials, and the exposure your specialty has had across the country as well as in your state and county. They also examine your, and your practice's, case history.

A few easy, low-cost avenues for mitigating med/mal risk and exposure are actually basic and require almost no extra effort.

## JEFF'S MED/MAL RISK MITIGATOR*

- Be kind to patients. Treat them like family. If you're unable to spend a great deal of time with each patient, make them feel as though you have. By this I mean include your extenders and other clinicians in the care cycle to assure that the patient feels their time was well spent and that you actually *cared* for them. *Listen to them and delight them.*

*This plan comes with no guarantees, whether stated, implied, or conceived in any way, shape, or form.*

- Be sure to have clinical care loops in place to assure closure on a patient's care. That is, if a test is ordered, assure that the test has been performed, that there is follow-up to the results of the test, that the appropriate referring MD has been contacted, and document the results/outcome.
- Anytime there is a therapy, treatment modality, or test, make sure the patient has been educated and has signed off on a consent. Make sure they understand the consent; don't just wave it under their nose and ask for a signature.
- Invest some money in staff training. A good, well-trained staff can help tremendously and is part of the care team. How *they* act toward and with the patients can also come into play in the patients' overall care experience. Staff can make or break you.

The med/mal climate has improved a bit in the recent past. But to give you an idea of the general situation, the Medical Group Management Association (MGMA) noted in their *MGMA Cost Survey* the med/mal increases realized by certain specialties during the last 12 years. MGMA pointed out that from 1997–2008 ob/gyn had med/mal costs per physician growing by about 39% from a median per physician of about $24,000 per year to almost $34,000 per year.[6] Cardiology, for that same time period, outpaced most specialties where median premiums per doc went from about $8,600 in 1997 to nearly $18,000 per physician in 2008,[7] a near 105% increase. Even though rates for both of these specialties have dropped a bit in the last few years, much of the increase occurred between 2002 and 2006. To mitigate some of these increases, some states have enacted tort reform, which has kept the cost of med/mal in check, relatively speaking. But you can see how your specialty and area of the country impact, and are impacted by, med/mal costs.[8]

In the interview process, I'd ask prospective employers if they have open claims. The worst they can do is tell you they don't wish to share that data/information. You might also inquire as to what they pay, per MD, for med/mal per year. Though the data out of context may mean nothing to you, as it varies from specialty to specialty and location to location, it will show your potential bosses that you are concerned about med/mal exposure and your questions might lead them to understand that you have a real interest about med/mal and the role exposure plays in the practice.

## BRINGING IT TOGETHER

Certainly these are not end-all, be-all questions. They do, however, cover a fair amount of the concerns you should be privy to when evaluating a position in a given geographic area.

The components of your search that we contemplate relative to practice type and area are not all-inclusive, but they do comprise a list that gets you closer to the right answer than many of your peers, who simply jump into this process without clear consideration as to where they want to be and the ramifications. The importance of these components depends on **your** values and the weight you place in each of these topics.

Also, it never hurts to ponder your outside interests. That is, does your area of choice have a good social component including active theater, outdoor activities, fine dining, and maybe a professional sports franchise or two? These are the extracurricular components that you'll need to merge into your process and be cognizant of to assure that your life outside of practice is equally as fulfilling as your life inside practice.

## PRACTICE TYPE

*Academic, Hospital-Based, or Private Practice*

It seems to me that the where-you-want-to-practice decision and the what-type-of-setting decision need be made almost simultaneously. That is, if you're into academic medicine and want to head to New Mexico, you might be limited in your career choices in that geographic area based on what academic centers are available in New Mexico and the rigorousness, or lack thereof, of their programs for your specialty. In your heart of hearts, if New Mexico is where you need to be, getting into private practice there should hold more opportunities for your given specialty. This may hold true for many areas in the country. If you love New Mexico and there are no academic opportunities available that you like (in your specialty), would you settle for private practice to be *where* you want to be?

Ok, now we'll first start with everyone letting down their guards and coming to grips with some realities.

Generally speaking, if you go into academic medicine, you can pretty safely expect to earn less than your private practice colleagues. But, you'll probably also work a little less (in terms of hours) and have a more reasonable life-schedule.

You may earn a bit less than your private practice colleagues because, as you may have surmised by now, we live in a risk/reward society. Private practitioners generally take on more risk than do their peers in the academic set and so the market should, and does, reward such behavior. But private practice also means more rigorous call, more demands on your private time and family time, and more effort in terms of hours. Sometimes, the job just doesn't end.

You may choose to become an employee of a hospital or hospital system. During the 1990s, many large hospitals gobbled up physician-owned practices with, in my opinion, the hope of obtaining, or keeping, referrals within the health system. Mind you, hospitals can't *demand* that employed MDs keep referrals in the system, since this is, well, illegal. However, I'm of the opinion that in some hospital strategic planner's mind there existed the glimmer of hope that "owned" MDs would keep their referrals within the system.

Many hospitals went on buying sprees, purchasing privately held medical practices. These deals were fraught with problems from the get-go when the hospitals, in many cases, overpaid for the groups and then hemorrhaged money because they guaranteed physicians' compensation and oftentimes overpaid the physicians. The unintended consequences were that once the practices were sold to the hospitals and the MDs were employees, the MDs now had different motivations. Gone were the responsibilities of trying to run a productive, efficient medical practice. Ushered in was the era of 9–5 medicine where MDs had neither a stake nor a risk in the practice's future. After all, it was no longer their business to run. And their backsides were no longer on the line. Physician compensation was no longer based on the effort of the physicians and efficiency of the operation. All in all, on its face, not a bad deal for the selling physicians. All in all, on its face, a massive wreck for the purchasing hospitals and hospital systems.

Put starkly and rather one-dimensionally, after the purchase, hospital administration tended to run the MD practice as they might have run a hospital. This model simply did not fit. Soon after, in the late 1990s, came a period of divestiture. Hospitals were anxious to shed money-losing medical practices. However, in the last few years some hospitals have once again begun acquiring private medical groups, but with greater attention to detail, a better sense of deals, and a smarter approach to negotiations. In fact, with continued decreasing reimbursements, many practices are now looking at expanded hospital relationships for protection.

In private practice, you are your own boss and you have a vested interest in what happens with and to that business. That is, it is your business and you can do with it as you please, within the realm of generally accepted business practices and laws. Revenues and subsequent profitability are directly related to your time spent in the office (though not necessarily proportionally so) so you can opt to take 2 months off a year or 2 weeks, but you must understand completely that your income may suffer or gain from those choices. And if you're in a group practice, chances of you taking 2 months off in your first year of practice are somewhere between zero and slim. Remember, there does exist the ever-present specter of peer pressure in private practice.

It seems an extension of common sense, though not a leap, to presume that most people reading this book are in, or will head into, private practice. Roughly 82% of you will end up in the private practice of medicine. Most physicians are either employed in private solo, group, or hospital-owned or -affiliated medical practices. With these settings come the inherent business concerns which we'll get into later. Generally, in an academic or hospital-based setting, you can look at your position as being employed by an institution where your main obligation is to show up to work and practice medicine. The institution handles a majority, if not all, of the paperwork apropos of the business, managerial headaches, and problems. There are no human resources issues for you to deal with. You simply punt your human resources problems up the chain of command to the hospital or academic center staff. Conversely, if you're in private practice, you need to deal with Suzy Q's incessant tardiness or Doctor Z's constant verbal assaults on other staff members. In private practice, you are running your own business and must deal with all of the issues that this encompasses.

After determining the practice setting you've chosen (academic, hospital-based, or private) and your desired area of the country, you may want to begin analyzing what type of group you'd like to be in. This section presupposes that you've selected a private medical practice. Are you looking to enter into a single-specialty, multi-specialty in a single classification (eg, ophthalmology), or a true multi-specialty group? Do you want to hang your own shingle and go it alone?

The type of medicine you want to practice and within what specialty or subspecialty may largely influence where you end up. If you want to work at the Cleveland Clinic, you'll either be in the greater Cleveland area, Toronto, Canada, or the greater Weston, Florida area.

The benefits of single-specialty, of course, are that all of the MDs and other clinicians "talk the same talk." You'll receive the benefit of counsel from your peers who understand the pathophysiology of your specialty and (one hopes) are up to date on clinical research and changes in the nuances of your specialty systems. As a new Fellow, access to these minds and communal experiences is priceless.

## DECISION PYRAMID — BUILDING ON THE FOUNDATION SETTING

*In what type of setting do you want to practice?*

*In what area of the country do you want to practice?*

Criteria for "Setting":
- Hospital-based, academic, private practice?
  - If private practice, group or solo?
    - If group, multi-specialty or single-specialty?
- Area opportunities for this set-up in your specialty?

## PRACTICE TYPE — SOLO VS GROUP

Basically, on the private practice side of medicine, practices can be broken down, in general terms, as either solo practice or group practice. The definition of solo speaks fairly well for itself.

Group practices are a different animal. Group practices can be a multi-specialty group comprised, quite literally, of specialties as incongruous as the day is long. For instance, you might have family practice, orthopedics, and ophthalmology in a multi-specialty group (though not likely).

**Solo group**: one physician; could have extenders, too, like nurse practitioners or physician assistants.

**Group practice**: multiple MDs, generally 3 or *more* (as per the AMA's definition of "group practice." This means one might surmise that a solo practice is up to 2 physicians!)

**Multi-specialty**: a sub-set of the group practice, I'd define this as either a group with more than one specialty or a group with associated specialties.

Examples:

**Tidewater Physician Management Group (TPMG)** – Tidewater is an amalgamation of nearly 60 physicians (not including extenders) treating patients in 24 locations with specialties ranging from internal medicine to sports med to gastroenterology to ob/gyn and ophthalmology. As you can see, this true multi-specialty group meets the definition.

http://www.tpmgpc.com

**Piedmont Health Care Group (PHC)** – nestled at the intersection of I-77 and I-40 just north of Charlotte, North Carolina, PHC employs 136 clinicians in multiple locations throughout the Piedmont region of North Carolina. As their Web site states:

"We have multiple convenient locations throughout Iredell and surrounding counties, including our convenient Urgent Care and Occupational Medicine facilities to better serve the needs of all our patients. Piedmont Health Care has more than 80 physicians offering a full range of medical services. With more than 20 specialties and primary care services, our patients have access to comprehensive medical care. With x-ray, CT, MRI, ultrasound and in-house laboratories, our patients have the option of receiving medical tests and procedures close to home. Just another reason Piedmont Health Care patients continue coming back to their physicians year after year and generation after generation."[9]

http://www.piedmonthealthcare.com/piedmont/index.asp

As you can see, in this definition of multi-specialty there are groups set up with a multitude of disease states handled under one practice "roof."

*Multi-specialty (in same functional area)*:

*Horizon Eye Care* – a group consisting of 22 clinicians (including ophthalmologists and optometrists) with 7 locations in and around Charlotte, North Carolina. Horizon is an ophthalmology group with a wide array of ophthalmology subspecialties. http://www.horizoneye.com/index.cfm/fuseaction/site.home.cfm

*Virginia Eye Institute (VEI)* – located in and around Richmond, Virginia, VEI has 31 clinicians (including ophthalmologists and optometrists) with 13 locations. VEI, again, is an ophthalmology group with a varied array of ophthalmology subspecialties.

http://www.vaeye.com/default.htm

*Midatlantic Cardiovascular* – this group has 69 clinicians practicing in 11 locations in and around the greater Baltimore area. Specializing in cardiovascular disease diagnosis and treatment, Midatlantic's clinicians cover a broad spectrum of treatment modalities in the specialty of cardiology.

http://www.midatlanticcardio.com/index.htm

As you have divined, the aforementioned groups are comprised of physicians with the same underlying specialty; for instance, an ophthalmology group with medical ophthalmology, surgical ophthalmology (eg, cataract and/or vision correction), cornea, retina, glaucoma specialists, and maybe a tumor and peds specialist for good measure.

*Single-specialty*: For our purposes, I'd look at single-specialty as a grouping of multiple physicians who practice the same "brand" of medicine. For instance, family practice or internal medicine.

Aspects, pros and cons, of each type of practice boiled down fairly simply:

Solo practice:

Pros:

- autonomy
- your own business
- flexibility of hours/workflow/patient schedule, etc

Cons:

- no group to work with; no one to bounce ideas off of
- your own business! The cost, debt, burden is on you
- when you're out on CME, vacation, etc, the place generates $0
- long, long hours; you're the sole breadwinner and so all of the pain falls on you. You see the patients *and* run the business in your copious free time (Good luck with that proposition.)

In any event, if you're looking to go solo, you'll be in for long hours. But for those of you who do better on your own, this'll do you some good. Make sure you find, and use, good counsel, in terms of accounting, management, and legal services.

Group practice:

Pros:

▪ see "Cons" for Solo practice above

Cons:

▪ see "Pros" for Solo practice above

When considering a group practice, there exist other little caveats worthy of con-templation. As you enter into a group setting, be it 4 MDs or 40 MDs, the politics and, dare I say, self-interest, can creep in. This can be, though not necessarily, pro-portional to the number of physicians in the group. I hasten to add *not necessarily* because if you're in a group of 4 MDs and you've one especially, we'll say . . . prickly . . . MD set in his/her ways, that can be just as bad as being in a 40-doc group with a mul-titude of troublemakers. The pain is predicated on the problem level associated with MD attitude.

Another thing to contemplate, both in group and solo doc endeavors, is this ques-tion: are there other outside businesses in which the practice has interests? For instance, is there a real estate holding company that you may want to buy into simul-taneously with your partnership buy in? If so, you'll need to understand all of the outside components as you move forward. This might come into play if you become a partner. (Eg, the practice rents office space from a limited liability company [LLC] owned primarily by the group.) You want to be sure that when it comes time to buy in to the medical practice, you at least have the opportunity to buy in to side corpo-rations that the company may have formed, the most common of which is the real estate holding company.

In terms of joining an MD who is currently solo, you'll want to ensure that the solo guy or gal is looking for a partner, if partnership is your ultimate goal. There might be a reason s/he is still solo, so I'd make sure to dig into the reasons, if ever so gently, for their continued solitude. Are they new to solo private practice and look-ing to add to their bustling business, or have they simply chased away all potential part-ners? Do they have a history of bringing along new associates only to cut them loose when it comes time to sign the dotted line of partnership? Do they hire new MDs and then, at the partnership doorstep, let them go? That does happen, just so you know. Is it unsavory? I think so.

These are things that require substantial investigation. You must make sure that, though the solo guy/gal is in charge, you at least have the opportunity to offer your input into the practice. You don't want to be a cog, but want instead to be recog-nized for the valuable contributor that you are. Will they pull all the strings or will they listen to your input? (In terms of medicine, if I were you, I'd not presuppose that you know too much about the business until you've had a few business meet-ings with the MD.)

## GROUP PRACTICE – SINGLE-SPECIALTY VS MULTI-SPECIALTY

This one's on you. It becomes more a matter of comfort than anything else. What I consider when writing this is the aspect of cohesion in a specialty. For instance, consider that you're in a multi-specialty practice, and you're the only ophthalmologist in that group. This might be sort of analogous to being the one-armed man in a paper hanging contest. In a single-specialty group, it may make sense to be comfortable in a group with other MDs who, though trained in different subspecs, are still cardiologists by training. And so that's helpful.

A multi-specialty group, on the other hand, may offer you the power in negotiating with payers for better reimbursement rates, but you may suffer in terms of camaraderie apropos of your specialty.

Again, there's no right or wrong answer, *per se*, just a matter of choice. But that choice could be limited by where, geographically, you're looking to practice. For instance, there are some cities in the country dominated by 1 or 2 large single-specialty groups. If you're interested in that area of the country, would you fit into a large group setting, assuming you're offered a job there? Or would you tough it out and try to compete either in a smaller group or on your own in the same city? Let me give you an example. I know of an area in the Southeast with the 2 major players in one specialty employing, between the 2 dominant groups, nearly 100 physicians. That's right, 100 physicians in 2 private practice medical groups practicing the same specialty. Pretty wild, no? Throw a third small group from that area into the mix (a group of merely 20 MDs) and you're looking at approximately 120 physicians in a city/area serving approximately 1.5 million people (as of 2006). And, for you guessing types out there, I'm not talking about Atlanta. So if you're heading to southeastern city X, could you function in a private practice group of 30–50 physicians? If not, would a smaller group in that area offer you what you want in terms of production and quality of life, even though you'd be on call every other night and every other weekend? Could you live in a smaller specialty group in a metro area where it's dog eat dog and where you will need to work harder to make a wage than you might otherwise make in rural Montana? There are a number of good reasons for being in a large group: group contracting, bargaining power, and leverage. Group purchasing (which affords the group certain economies of scale) and a better call schedule. But there are also downsides, such as being a small fish in a big pond.

## DECISION PYRAMID – GROUP COMPOSITION

- Private practice
  - Group or solo
    — If group, multi-specialty or single-specialty?
      ◆ If multi-specialty, pure multi-spec or specialty-related?

- Area opportunities in your specialty and group setting

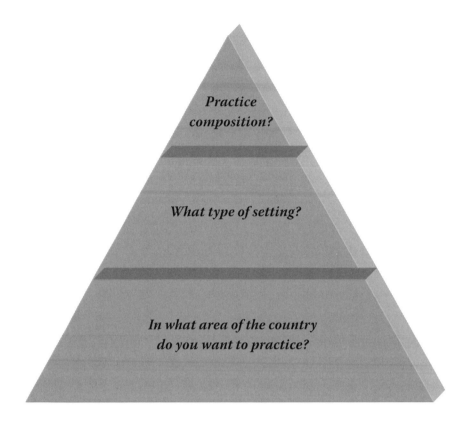

## TOPPING OFF THE PYRAMID

Built on quasi-logical components, the preceding was a non-exhaustive list of what you'll want to look at in your job search. Some of the components are intertwined with others adding, perhaps, some weight to their value in the decision-making process. Most are not mutually exclusive, but you probably cannot have all in equal shares (eg, you cannot get 100% of each component you're searching for) and you will need to decide which components you're willing to give a little on to get more of something else. You'll need to define what your priorities are that will ultimately give you the quality of life you are looking for and that will satisfactorily launch your career on the right path. Take none of them in a vacuum, but instead evaluate all of them, in order of importance to you, in moving forward in your search.

Did you notice how *my* key components did *not* include you joining practice with your friends from med school? That's because, though you may have a wondrous life with them outside of work if you're in the same practice, if you hate your job, you'll hate your life, and you may ultimately foster some resentment toward the friend who assisted you into the quagmire, I mean predicament, you find yourself in. It's that simple. So find a practice you can live in and grow with, regardless of whether or not your friends are there.

Remember, the pyramid was built to delineate some structural basics and items to ponder for your successful job search. The cap of the pyramid is all the detail we'll dig into further in the book, including the business side of things.

## SHOW ME THE JOB: LOCATING THE RIGHT JOB— RECRUITERS, BUDDIES, AND PALS

There are decidedly different avenues for a clinician to find the right job. Included on that road are the professional recruiters who are generally either retained or contingency fee-based.

For the most part, retained firms might be more of the norm for a health system or hospital, as they might have many open searches throughout the year and need a company, or multiple companies, searching on their behalf full time to fill their open physician slots. Private practices, however, might have a finite need, 1 or 2 slots to fill, that are very specific and don't require an ongoing retained relationship with a recruiter. In these instances, the practice might choose to use a contingency fee-based recruiter. Contingency agreements are usually for the duration of a search, but can be for an ongoing relationship where the agreement is signed and in effect every time a practice has a physician need to fill.

These 2 forms of agreement are what they seem: a retained search is where a firm is paid to find a candidate. A contingency agreement is where the recruiter is not paid until after the candidate is delivered, meaning payment is contingent upon the deal coming to fruition. It's not unheard of in a contingency agreement for a recruiter to place a candidate and receive a majority, if not all, of their fee after the placement. Some caveats built into the contingency agreement may allow for the practice to recoup some of its money if a candidate does not last on the job for 6 months or a year.

Recruiters are a good way to go in your search. Since it's their business, many recruiters have their ears to the ground and have a feel for what jobs are out there. They'll do a great deal of the legwork for you. There are also recruiters who work in subspecialties. They have their business ears to the ground hunting out, either nationally or regionally, certain jobs for certain specialties. So, if you are in a specialty with limited spots available, these recruiters might offer an even more acute awareness of certain opportunities throughout the country. A recruiter can help cut down on the paperwork and minimize the length of the search process. And it's a good business for them, when they make a hit. In some specialties, a recruiter will garner $18,000–$30,000 to land *one* physician for a practice. Not bad, if you consider it. But on the recruiter side of the business, that endeavor is dog eat dog and fairly arduous.

Lastly, so you know, most recruiters work for the searching physician group, which means the hiring practice will pay the finder's fee. If a recruiter asks for a fee from you, run, don't walk, to the nearest door or away from the nearest Internet connection. Though I've never seen this scenario, you can rest assured that folks like these are not looking out for you. It's the same theory in writing: if an agent wants money from you up front, they're in it for them, not you.

You may want to contact your associates to determine who and what firms they've used in the past apropos of recruiters.

## THE "FRIENDS NETWORK"

At some point in your job search, you may very well have a recruiter working for you in addition to getting information from an associate or friend via word of mouth. This can be very effective and costs neither party anything in terms of placement. Job searches via word of mouth can be very productive. You may also try looking via your specialty society, as most have active placement pages on their Web sites and throwaways. These serve as fertile locations to chase down available positions within your specialty. Another source of job leads in your specialty may be the state medical society in a state you've pondered, or your specialty society state chapter, if they have one. (Eg, the American College of Cardiology has several state chapters.)

## NOW, LAND YOUR IDEAL GROUP

So you've determined where you want to be geographically, what type of group you're looking for, you've reviewed the payer mix, and you've figured out how many specialists there are . . . or you've done none of these things and tossed caution to the wind. Your next job, even given these attributes of your search, might not be the end all, be all for you. It might not be the last stop on your career continuum, but hopefully you've performed your due diligence and think you've selected an area and practice site that suits both your, and your significant other's, needs.

Now it's time to begin flipping over the rocks. Make sure that you have your *curriculum vitae* (CV) in order. Ensure that it lists your education and recent experience leading the way, along with where you attended school, publications, studies, research, etc. **Never** put your social security number on your CV and, really, there's no need to put personal interests or family information on your CV. No one cares that your wife was born in Palo Alto or that you have 3 kids: Maggie, Chris, and Fred. The group is not hiring your family, and though your familial situation is interesting, it's not of concern to the group you're courting. The CV should serve as an aperitif in getting your foot in the door. If you take a step toward the altar of contractual matrimony, you can then cover your interests over a nice refined recruiting dinner. Remember, there is no need for the hiring practice to know about your family, and technically, they have no legal right to inquire (many hiring MDs do not know this).

Once you have your CV well in hand, *you* need to begin contacting groups, whether they're looking for you or not, to let them know that you're out there and you have an interest.

There's plenty of demand for good physicians and, as I've said, you should not need to pay for the privilege of using a recruiter; they should be paid by a group for what *you* bring to the table. Demand for health care is on the rise as the population ages and the supply of physicians is not expected to meet that demand.

Then it's off to the races. Though your CV does not need to be pristine (as many MDs read for content vs style), it should be presentable. After all, you're getting ready for the big dance. You're prospectively looking at a group for a second marriage. Your first impression with the parents should be a good one. Make it count and stand out.

As an aside, as a business person, I'm still interested in spelling, grammar, some punctuation. So I'm looking to see that you have some sort of a mastery of the English language. But that's me. I think everyone I hire should have some sort of proficiency in English. Now, as an aside to that aside, if you're dealing with a large group, whether single-spec or multi-spec, your chances are good that the head of that ship (from a business perspective) is a PhD, an MBA, an MHA, a JD, or some combination thereof. In more advanced practices (advanced is defined as groups with a prototypical business structure), the folks running the ship most likely will see and pass your resume on to a reviewing committee or some other body assigned with reviewing CVs. That means that a layman like me will take a look at what you submit and *may* be in a position to give you the thumbs down from the get-go. Is that fair? No, as we're not clinicians. Does that matter? No, it does not.

When you identify a practice to go after, I'd make some cold calls to determine if there's a standing search committee within the practice or, if the group is small, a lead doc to whom you could send your CV. In larger groups, I'd copy the administrator, if you can garner his or her name. Some administrators are more in touch with the clinical recruiting needs of the practice than are their physician-bosses and so an astute administrator might just see a good CV for a very defined business need within the group. (Think a cardiology group looking for an EP guy or gal to round out their cardiology continuum of care.)

Another source, of course, is your friends, as discussed previously. You've probably got some friends who finished a year or 2 ahead of you and are now out in the real world. They might know of positions that are available, have a keen understanding of what compensation might look like, and can be key to getting you in the door.

You should aggressively go after the groups you have an interest in. As I've said, even if they are not advertising for a position, it is worth submitting your CV to them.

It shows interest, motivation, and initiative. And you never know when they might pull out your CV and give you a call.

And remember this: if a group is interested in interviewing you, the cost of the process is borne by *them,* not you. They should provide sufficient cash to pay for your expenses including, but not limited to: reasonable air travel, a rental car, a hotel, and minor miscellaneous items like tolls, etc. But, worth noting, don't tuck in a bunch of miscellaneous garbage on the receipts you submit for reimbursement. Keep your expenses to what you've done in association with the recruiting trip. When I, or someone like me, review those expenses before we make payment, exaggerated or over inflated expenses are a pretty darned good red flag for us. How? Well, if you're willing to cheat on your expenses during a recruitment trip, what the heck else might you cheat on?

The way the process will probably go is you will make your flight reservations and other travel arrangements. Pay for those services, then keep your receipts and turn them in after your recruiting trip. I have also seen some groups make the arrangements for the interviewee. This is fine, as you don't need to charge your trip, but I like to let the visiting MD do that stuff so that s/he can arrange the trip based on their needs and time constraints.

## COMPENSATION

We'll now take a leap. You're employable (good for you), and someone actually has an interest in you (even better!). The stars are aligned and you feel like you've waltzed gingerly into a perfect job fit.

When you get in with your group, there'll be a myriad of questions to ask and avoid. As a reformed interviewer of MDs, I feel as though I know a few of those. You can find some of those in the appendix of this book.

Now that you've decided to dance with this group, and take steps toward your second marriage, it's time to figure out what you're worth. How do you know what you're worth to the group? Well, you've done your research on the area in terms of the specialty demand, you know how many docs there are out there and you have an idea of the possible patient demographics; you know that you are worth a good bit to the group (or not). But first, you need a baseline. A jumping-off point, if you will, to know how much above or beyond a reasonable salary you should go.

You're well on your way, staking territory that you're interested in, creating a log of the submissions of your CVs, follow-up timeframes, key contacts, and the like. You're showing a real interest in getting in the door. I'd suggest you'll need a very confident understanding about what you might earn in your first year out. Let's look at some of the basics.

## WHAT DO PHYSICIANS IN YOUR SPECIALTY MAKE?

The $64,000 question and the 800-pound gorilla, all wrapped into 2 overly used metaphors. Ostensibly, you got into health care to make a difference, for the scientific and academic pursuit inherent in advancing your chosen field, for helping people live better lives via the delicate balance of art and science, and for making a difference to mankind's overall well-being. (I'm serious here, so no snickering.) But also, you have to get paid for what you do. In my opinion, you should be paid fairly. Do you deserve an NFL salary? Probably. Will you get one? I know you wouldn't ask for that with a straight face! But I've always labored under some Pollyanna-ish belief that folks who are good at what they do should, by market drivers, make a better wage than those folks who stink at what they do. Call me crazy.

That said, some pragmatic and basic tenets of economics come into play when you're looking at prospective positions and areas. Please review page 4:

1. How many MDs are there in your chosen area?
2. What is the payer mix? (There it is again.)

### HOW MANY MDs

Econ 101, supply and demand. The more physicians per patient in an area *may* mean lower compensation for MDs in that area. Again, more supply means the market may reward less (eg, there is no scarcity of physicians). Add to that mix a healthy dose of extenders (physician assistants and nurse practitioners) and that may or may not negatively impact compensation. If you're in an area of low competition, or your practice is the dominant group in the area, available compensation may end up being on the higher end for your specialty.

### PAYER MIX

This harkens back to our discussion about who pays what in your geographic area of choice. For instance, if Medicare is your best payer, compensation rates for clinicians *could* be lower.

### SOURCES AND SOURCES

So, it all depends. There are professional associations out there that aggregate data on physician productivity and compensation. They will not give up the information for free, as you might imagine, so be prepared to pay what should be a nominal fee to access the data.

In my opinion, the dominant group vis-à-vis practice management is the Medical Group Management Association (MGMA), probably the largest medical management association in the country, boasting approximately 21,000 members. In the practice management arena, the MGMA might be analogous to the AMA for medicine; a big umbrella for all specialties. Then, within the MGMA there are subspecialty affiliations, such as the cardiothoracic surgery/cardiology assembly (CSCA) or the ophthalmology assembly (OA). Also, some of the medical specialty societies have practice management components whose value and veracity of data (in terms of practice management) can be touchy, depending on the number of responses they receive from queried individuals. The MGMA is an organization with resources and a history in medical practice management dating back to 1929. They perform a variety of surveys annually. For instance, for their 2009 Physician Compensation Survey (reflecting 2008 data) they purported an estimated 2,246 returned surveys, according to William F. Jessee, MD, FACMPE, (Fellow of the American College of Medical Practice Executives) President and CEO. All things being equal, that type of response might be, on its face, of some value. But if you're an endocrinologist, how do you know how many endocrinologists submitted data? As scientists, you know the more data, the better. Same applies to practice management data. So if only 2 endocrinologists submitted data, and one MD's salary was $1,000,000 and the other MD made $100,000, you have a very bizarre range and final result that has just about as much value as a fishing pole on a prairie. You may want to investigate little offshoot subspecialty groups that have evolved over the years and have aggregated data on their own. In some subspecialties, like cardiology, there exists a very rich repository of data that has grown over time. Generally speaking, though, the MGMA's data is pretty good, but its specialty and region-specific stuff, in my humble opinion, leaves a little something to be desired, depending on the number of respondents. But it is definitely a great starting point.

The MGMA also offers academic compensation surveys.

Other organizations specializing in medical practice management include the American Medical Group Association (AMGA). The AMGA has a slightly different take on practice management than does the MGMA, according to its mission statement, and it " . . . advocates for the multispecialty medical group model of health care delivery and for the patients served by medical groups, through innovation and information sharing, benchmarking, leadership development, and continuous striving to improve patient care."[10]

Founded in the late 1940s, it too focuses on the medical practice setting, looking mainly at a multi-specialty delivery model.

Additionally, there exist hospital-based organizations specializing in hospital-related vs private medical practice data. Consultants and management advisors in your specialty, or well-versed generalists, should have a good feel for what you might expect for a starting salary.

You can also turn to your friends, but they often offer anecdotal information that I've found, over my time in this business, is not so accurate. Some people, for whatever reason, jack up their comp and vacation, I guess to show off to their friends. Who knows?

In any event, you know the supply and demand in your market of choice. You understand some of the basics. Given that data and understanding, two components should resonate and those are that you neither want to be greedy nor sell yourself too short. So you need to find balance.

Here's the tricky part. You've just left Fellowship and have, aside from killing yourself, been pulling in a modest $35,000–$ 40,000 a year while racking up a healthy 6-figure student loan debt obligation. Basically, as a full-time employee, your $35K per year would boil down to about $16.83/hour or, more precisely, $16.8269. To put that into perspective, in ophthalmology, most first-level certified technicians (Certified Ophthalmic Assistants [COAs]) make $14–$18/hour, depending on the region of the country and their experience. And my hourly rate calculations presume you **only** worked what's considered a normal work year (eg, 40 hours per week). Did you do that during Fellowship? If not, you may have made less than $16.83/hour! (Just so you know, at the time of this writing, Congress had approved a minimum wage increase from $5.85 in the summer of 2007 to a whopping $7.25/hour as of 2009. As a Fellow, did you make at least the minimum wage?)

That said, in looking at your first job, an offer of $100,000 might sound very enticing. It beats the heck out of $35,000 a year, right? But how does that sound apropos of the **value** of the job? What do you bring to the table relative to that job? Anything special? (I know, you've made it through med school and all the rigors and you're special. Let's tuck that knowledge in our back pocket, shall we?) Or will you be a cog in the wheel? Are you, as we tactfully call it, a shelf stocker? Or is there sufficient competition in the area to warrant you garnering a slightly, maybe even significantly, higher salary?

Let's boil that down just a bit. How much might you expect to generate in revenue for the business? How many new patients does the group you're dancing with see in a year and per MD? How much ancillary business is there? Are there other businesses that you might be a party to? Do you prime the pump (eg, are you simply seeing patients whilst others perform surgeries, both minor and major)?

Does the job pay $100,000/year to new Fellows just coming out or $250,000? As a shameless plug, I'd check with a management advisor to ascertain what one might expect to make in that area. This exercise, though not without a nominal cost (probably not more than $250) would be worth the investment if you look at it in terms of making $250,000 vs $200,000 per year. (In other words, a $50,000 return on your $250 investment in the advisor—a 20,000% return.)

How do you know what you bring to the practice? Well, let us presume that you might run a basic bell curve in your visits during a year. I'm a fairly conservative guy when it comes to the nuts and bolts, so I'd just assume, for argument's sake, that you will do nothing but see patients. You'll perform no tests, you'll offer no surgeries. You'll just see patients every day you work in the practice. As you know, a Gaussian function is a basic "normal" distribution curve. So we'll presume that you will have this model, seeing a small number of level 1 Current Procedural Terminology (CPT®) visits, a few more level 2 CPT® visits, an even higher number of level 3, and then diminishing in the number of level 4 and 5 CPT® codes billed. Of course, you'll need to know what CPT®s you might bill in your specialty. However, I'll keep the example simple. Our given assumptions are these, for simplicity's sake:

1. The group you're joining has a very definite demand for a new physician. (Put differently, if you are not seeing a bunch of patients when you join, they added you for no apparent reason.)

2. Let's say that you're a primary care physician in Atlanta, Georgia, and that you will bill only new patient visits, codes 99201–99205[11] on new patients and codes 99211–99215[12] on rechecks. We will bill no consult codes (which tend to reimburse a bit higher due to their nature and complexity) and we assume that you and your group "par," or participate with Medicare, which also offers you an eensey-weensy premium for participating in the program. Since, generally speaking, Medicare and Medicaid will be your worst payers (sorry Florida, I know that's not true for many of you) we'll assume safe Medicare rates. We would then multiply the number of expected patient visits for each CPT® code with the corresponding payment for each code, yielding a conservative guesstimate of what you might reasonably be expected to generate, ***solely*** in new patient and recheck visits.

3. All you see is Medicare patients. Medicare rates are known throughout the country, regardless of where you practice. Using Medicare as an example offers you definitive knowledge of reimbursement.

4. We'll assume you see 25 patients each day, 20% of whom might be new patients. So you'll have 5 new patients and 20 rechecks daily. We'll then spread those out as a normal distribution curve. (see Exhibit 4 on page 29)

5. You will have 25 days off (5 weeks of combined vacation and CME) so you'll work 47 weeks out of the 52 per year.
   The results of our little exercise are displayed in Exhibit 2.

As you can see, in your "typical" week in the trenches, being reimbursed no better than Medicare rates for greater Atlanta, based on the above assumptions, you might expect to generate $9,050.55 in revenue. Remember, though, this is built on the assumption that you're going great guns and seeing 25 patients per day. For good measure, let's

**EXHIBIT 2.**

| | Assumes 5 weeks (25 days) off per year for V/CME | | | | | |
|---|---|---|---|---|---|---|
| | | | | | | |
| | Total daily patient visits: | | | 25 | | |
| | NP: | | | 5 | | |
| | Rechecks: | | | 20 | | |
| | | | | | | |
| | Bell Curve of Visits– Annual Gaussian Distribution | | | | | |
| Annual | | | | | | |
| 99201 | 99202 | 99203 | 99204 | 99205 | CPT® Code(s) | |
| 0 | 235 | 705 | 235 | 0 | Patient visits | |
| | | | | | | |
| 99211 | 99212 | 99213 | 99214 | 99215 | CPT® Code(s) | |
| 705 | 940 | 1410 | 940 | 705 | Patient visits | |
| | | | | | | |
| Annual revenue | | | | | | |
| Atlanta | | | | | | |
| Annual | | | | | | |
| 99201 | 99202 | 99203 | 99204 | 99205 | | |
| $ - | $15,014.15 | $65,170.20 | $33,496.90 | $ - | | |
| | | | | | | Per working week (47) |
| 99211 | 99212 | 99213 | 99214 | 99215 | | |
| $13,338.60 | $35,146.60 | $87,152.10 | $87,467.00 | $88,590.30 | $425,375.85 | $9,050.55 |

take a look at geographic disparities. Medicare pays you differently in different areas of the country. We'll visit the reasons for this fact later in the book.

For now, I dropped in the revenues that the same patient mix and assumptions would generate if you were seeing patients in the Richmond, Virginia area (Exhibit 3).

As you can see, the same mix of patients provides $17,251.35 *less* revenue in Richmond than it does in Atlanta. Atlanta is reimbursed higher by Medicare, ostensibly because of the greater cost of doing business in metro Atlanta.

In any event, in Atlanta, if you have 5 weeks off per year, that equates to roughly $425,375.85 in revenue generated by you for a calendar year. Not so bad. This offers

**EXHIBIT 3.**

| Richmond, VA | | | | | | |
|---|---|---|---|---|---|---|
| 99201 | 99202 | 99203 | 99204 | 99205 | | |
| $ – | $14,363.20 | $62,399.55 | $32,218.50 | $ – | | Per working week (47) |
| 99211 | 99212 | 99213 | 99214 | 99215 | | |
| $12,633.60 | $33,492.20 | $83,711.70 | $84,064.20 | $85,241.55 | $408,124.50 | $8,683.50 |
| | | | | | | |
| | Diff between Richmond and Atlanta— Same work & # of pts seen. | | | $-17,251.35 | | |

you a glimpse into what you might generate in 1 year of a full patient load. Assuming the practice you're interviewing with has a 50% overhead ratio which, as an employee would include your salary, you return about $212,687.93 ($425,375.85 x .50) to the practice.

What the heck did we just accomplish? Well, we displayed the revenue you might generate if you did nothing but see Medicare patients in a primary care-type setting with a 50% overhead ratio. And this offers you an idea of a baseline for your revenue generation for a full year. What does this get you, in terms of negotiation? Maybe nothing, again, depending on the clinician competition in the area, the practice's need for new clinicians based on patient demands, and your personal needs and desires. But it might offer you some bargaining leverage in negotiating either your salary or total compensation package and, at the very least, offer you a baseline relative to what you might generate doing nothing but seeing patients and getting reimbursed at Medicare's rates.

Keep in mind, the key to this exercise and its veracity is tied into the actual practice need for a new clinician. Is there pent-up patient demand for a new MD? Put differently, are there too many patients for the current MDs of the practice to see?

Also, in Exhibit 4, you can see the bell distribution for 25 patients daily based on the facts above.

## JEFF, GIVE ME THE BOTTOM LINE

Dr X, there is no magic bullet. You'll learn a great deal as you go along in this business and one of the things you'll determine is that there generally is not a definite right or wrong answer, particularly when dealing with physicians. Ultimately, the salary, total compensation, and path-to-partnership discussions boil down to effective negotiation and coming to terms with a deal each party can live with, as with any negotiation.

But do understand this, too. When looking for a position, there is usually a fairly acceptable compensation rate or range. As you evaluate positions and aggregate com-

**EXHIBIT 4**

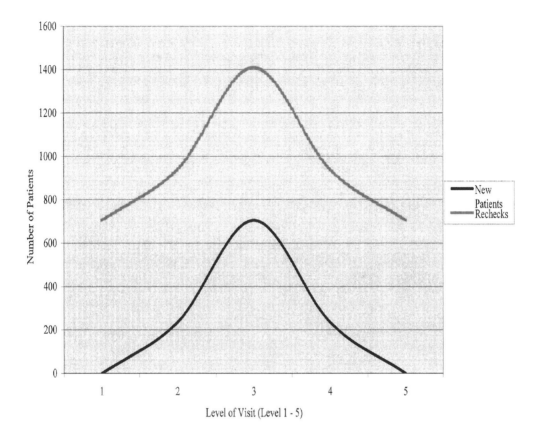

Normal distribution of visits

pensation figures, take pains to understand anomalies in the compensation data. If the comp package is too high, might that be an indication of a massive and burdensome call schedule for the new associates? If compensation is too low, might the group be struggling with debt obligations or might the new physicians be propping up older docs who've slowed down, are working less, and taking less call? These outliers, though not deal breakers, do require further investigation and analysis before you jump in.

My advice to you is to understand what you want, shoot for the stars, but know what you'd be happy with and keep your expectations planted on *terra firma*. In any event, I think I've armed you with some tools and information that might better enable you to arrive at a reasonable compensation rate that pays you slightly more than an ophthalmic technician might make.

Author's note: this book, as a practical resource, is hereafter interspersed with the occasional real-world anecdote. All anecdotes are denoted by the preceding phrase ***Fun/Educational Anecdote Number X.*** Now onward and upward with:

## FUN/EDUCATIONAL ANECDOTE NUMBER 1

Please be reasonable in your expectations and honest in your introspection. I'll never forget the specialist I interviewed after she had just finished Fellowship who expected a starting salary somewhere around $500,000 per year. Now, though that may be feasible in some areas of the country and in some specialties and/or subspecialties, that is the exception and not the rule in first year comp. Needless to say, we opted not to continue our discussions with that physician and I'm sure she found a home somewhere else (but I can almost guarantee not at that money) and we ended up landing a seasoned, reasonable clinician who, it turned out, was worth his weight in gold.

Understanding what you might generate, even if overly conservative, might be a worthwhile exercise.

One last parting shot across the bow: it's prudent to make sure that if you're relying on your buddies to let you know what to ask for in salary, be advised that their salary may be an amalgamation of total compensation, which may include profit sharing, vacation, CME, and travel allowances. Always make apples-to-apples comparisons. Salary is not total compensation.

## TYPE OF ORGANIZATION

There are a couple of corporate structures in terms of tax status and treatment that you'll hear about in the medical community. Each has its pluses and minuses, but many private practices are either organized as Professional Corporations ("S" or "C" [subchapter S or subchapter C of the IRS code) or as LLCs (limited liability companies). You'll see these most frequently. How the corporation's tax structure has been set impacts the tax effect on the owners, so it'd be fairly prudent for you, at some time during your employment and prior to partnership, to understand the corporation's tax structure, in order to give you a feel of how it might impact you, personally, when you become partner.

I am not an accountant, so I won't entertain the idea of offering you specifics about what is right/wrong with each type of organization. What I will tell you is the following.

## PROFESSIONAL CORPORATION

A professional corporation (PC) is organized as either a subchapter S or a subchapter C entity. In a "C Corp," all income must be paid out in salary or bonus by December 31 of the current year. If it is not, the company must pay corporate income tax. The physicians involved in this structure, like staff, receive a paycheck and are paid on the same schedule as employees. This means, for the most part, that all employees of the company receive their checks together, normally every 2 weeks, which equates to 26 pay periods during the year. The owners of the corporation, the partners, set the rules and can determine pay out of special (and other) bonuses. So normally, all income is paid out. There generally are no retained earnings (eg, money left over for projects). Instead, most projects are financed over time with the financing entity like a bank. Rather than receive draws, each owner (shareholder) receives a salary and/or bonus from which taxes are deducted at time of payment. At some point before January 31 of the next year, each physician receives a W-2 form that includes all salary and tax data for the preceding year. The effect of this is that physician taxes are paid with each paycheck, and in most cases the need for quarterly tax estimates is eliminated. "C Corps" are taxed at both a corporate and shareholder level. "S Corps" allow all income to be passed through to shareholders so they are taxed only once.

An LLC is considered, for tax purposes, to be a partnership. So all income, taxes, and deductions are passed through to the partners (or members) individually, making each partner liable for his or her pro rata share of deductions, depending upon ownership. Annually, partners are issued a K-1 instead of a W-2 summary. In an LLC, all income does not necessarily have to be paid out by year's end. That is a decision the owners can make. Partners are taxed on their share of profit, which is practice receipts and revenues minus expenses incurred while running the practice. Whether or not cash remains in the practice, it is taxed on that year's personal income tax return for each partner. So, you could retain earnings to begin a project because those dollars, whether you reinvest them or pay them out, are taxable. A K-1 is issued to let the partners know how much to include on their tax return. So, in a PC you would be taxed on the W-2 wages; in the LLC you are taxed on the amount of income attributed to each partner that *could be* withdrawn, since that money is considered earned. In an "S Corp", you could receive a W-2 *and* a K-1.

Both the PC and LLC forms of practice work. The choice boils down more to a question of which entity works best for a group. Anecdotally, many large medical groups operate in professional corporation form.

For more pros/cons about either practice structure, contact an accountant and, if possible, one who has dealt with medical practice structures. Dazzle him/her with your *facile* understanding of PCs and LLCs, and ask his/her opinion. Most will talk to you for free as they look to you as a potential big earner (and therewith prospective business) client.

## THE INTERVIEW PROCESS

Once you've selected your geography, the type of medical group you're interested in, prepared your CV, divined the handful of groups you're going to market yourself to, and figured an idea of the revenue you might generate, it's time to begin the interview process. I'd suggest you go to as many interviews as possible, even with the groups on your list that may not be your highest ranked. The reason is you grow from the experience, you get to see a variety of different operations, and you attain a familiarity and comfort with the interview process; a process which says a great deal about the group. Plus, you'll be reimbursed for the trips and their associated expenses. Remember, you don't need to jump at the first thing you see. Consider your options and know that if the group is truly interested in you as a new associate, there'll probably be another dinner and house-hunting trip in your future.

On the big day, you'll have on your neatest dark suit, a crisp white shirt, a red power tie, perhaps, or a pretty floral dress or pantsuit. I'll leave gender differences and style choices up to the individual relative to clothing selection germane to them.

Your interview exposure to the group begins with this, simply enough: the vibe. You'll know it when you feel it, and you'll need to know what goes on underneath the interview, under the cutesy veneer. In other words, let's face it, when you're interviewing, all parties are on their best behavior. That means all the skeletons will be tucked neatly away, periodicals and throwaways stacked crisply in front of them, and the interviewers will have on their best Sunday dress. You're all there for show, a dance around the prospect of your employment.

You'll need to cut through the vacuous interview niceties and get a feel for who's where and who does what. Which MDs are included in the interview process? The managing partner? An MD you'll work with in a satellite office, ostensibly someone you'll need to be tight with? Or is there, in a larger group, an interviewing body that will pass you around, take you to dinner, and generally pass judgment?

Watch the dynamic of the interviewing physicians. Learn who the key MDs in the group are and what positions they hold. Are the senior MDs there? Do the young guys bite their tongues in the presence of the older guys? Or does everyone seem to say what's on his/her mind, painfully free to speak his/her mind sans the fear of retribution? Do the physicians, generally, get along well? Do the partners, more specifically, get along well? (A means to that answer, outside of an overt smack to the head, is a question couched like *Do you do anything outside of the office with your partners?*" or "*What activities do you and your partners do outside of the office?*")

If catching that vibe is on the tips of your fingers, request to interview *each* partner, or, if a large group, a fair number of partners. Talk to them about the group, about direction, about where they see things going in the next year. Inquire about the following 2–5 years. And, though a bit of a stretch, ask them where they see the group in 10 years. Dance delicately around the partnership and the numbers. Talk about the group's history, find out about the longevity of MDs, and then ask the interviewing partner what he or she thinks about their partners. Ask them about group cohesion. Remember this, and never forget it during the process. This is your second marriage. These are the people who very well may hold the keys to your career in their hands. And these are the people you'll need to be willing to lie down in traffic for, as they would (one hopes) for you. Once you become partner, extracting yourself from the group may very well be as complicated, or more complicated, than extracting yourself from a marriage. So ask the questions you need to, and make sure you find balance between "need to know" for the interview and "none of your business" for other things. The interviewing doctors should not, technically, ask you personal lifestyle-related questions. You should keep your questions practice-centric and focused on the partnership and the job at hand. Then you'll both be on the right track.

These questions are key. The interactions when you meet the group can be indicative and help you gain a vibe, the true vibe, on the energy of the practice. Generally, I'd separate gut from reason on this and let my gut win that battle. As with test taking, your first instinct is usually your best.

## FUN/EDUCATIONAL ANECDOTE NUMBER 2

An associate passed on the following anecdote. It was a simple, direct to the point anecdote that said it all in one simple sentence. While interviewing for a job as an administrator, an angry MD interviewing the candidate said (paraphrasing), "My partners are out to get me." Needless to say, the interviewee did not pursue that job any further as he received, fairly bluntly, the wrong vibe and determined in short order that group cohesion. . . . wasn't.

Will you be able to tell, during the interview process, what the group cohesion looks like? Will there be a glaring example similar to that in *Fun/Educational Anecdote Number 2*?

Honestly, probably not. At first blush, you may not notice any of these social cues. You'll be a racing bundle of caffeine and adrenaline hopping from MD to MD on a string of nervous energy, and they'll be preoccupied with the interviewing process and trying to ponder how their day with patients is going to look, so your initial vibe may be fleeting. If it's not, if you sense something amiss right off the bat, identify an egress with due haste.

Remember, you might feel discomfited by these questions, but this is a dynamic, two-way process. *You're* interviewing *them*, too. And this is something you need to know. The more you hold back in this process, the less you'll know. The less you know, the more you harm yourself, and ultimately, the group, as you'll be a miserable sop trying to figure out how to get out of the group and maybe even, subconsciously, trying to subvert the very thing you once coveted: partnership.

Thoughts to ponder (and questions to punt to the MD partners) during the interview process:

- How do you get along with your partners?
- What are the work habits of the group?
- Is there a penalty committee, or overall management committee, in place?

## NEW VS OLD

With physicians I've interviewed of late, I've noted a marked difference in disposition vis-à-vis their predecessors. Younger MDs these days don't define themselves as physicians, but more as dads, husbands, wives, and mothers who practice medicine. This is a demarcation heretofore unseen and decidedly different from the way things were 20, maybe as few as 10 years ago, when a physician defined himself by the arduous hours invested in his career and seemingly gauged his progress by the time lost with his family. The physician of today seems to see the benefits of working hard during the work week, making a decent wage, and spending valuable time with his family. As someone wiser than me once said, no one is going to look at you in the casket and say, "he was the best administrator I've ever met." (Plug in "doctor" where you see "administrator" and you'll get the picture.) If they do, then I personally feel that I'd taken a serious sidestep and missed out on my priorities in life, lost my balance. Don't get me wrong, working hard is fun, good, liberating, and empowering. You derive a certain sense of satisfaction in a job well done. You feel a tangible sense of accomplishment, a palpable feeling of value, but when all is said and done, no matter how much you love your job, your job will never love you back. Remember that phrase: your job will *never* love you back.

There can exist the problem of older physicians resenting younger MDs and their "lack of dedication" to the business and the practice of medicine. I'd suggest to you that nothing could be further from the truth. Physicians today are no less interested in delivering quality patient care and the best patient outcomes, but MDs today just beginning practice have an entirely different climate that they're entering and so their professional needs, demands, and desires have shifted to accommodate that and their personal needs.

Apropos of age, other questions of import are the median and mean ages of the physicians. If the ages are fairly high, do you foresee a slowdown or difference in call coverage, work ethic, etc? If so, has that been addressed in the corporate documents and have allowances been made to replace any slowing physicians? That could come into play. You might end up being the dumping ground for the grunt work as a seasoned MD slows down, reduces calls, and yet receives all of the perks a senior guy/gal feels entitled to. Are you going to be the guy or gal who is perpetually there after hours reading tests or dictating while all the other MDs have hit the golf course?

Additionally, one caveat new MDs tend to miss is whether or not the senior guys have senior protections. Essentially, senior protections are little caveats placed in the partner contracts that oftentimes insulate a handful of senior guys from getting cut from the group by anyone other than other senior guys with senior protections. For instance, if Drs 1, 2, and 3 are senior, and docs 4–10 are junior, even if there's a coup afoot by the young guys, the only way to oust an "old" (read Drs 1–3) guy is for 2 of the 3 senior guys to dump the third. Of course, this is without cause or breaking of the law. That goes without saying.

After your first interview, if everyone is still in love and the courting group has asked for your hand, if you'll excuse the overused metaphor, you'll want to know, in great detail, what the partnership track is. For instance, do you buy in after year 1 of employment? And if so, is this purely a cash transaction or is it a graduated payment? Do you buy stock in the company at a fixed price? These are important questions that are worth broaching, even if only peripherally, to give you an understanding of what happens *after* you've been an employee. Questions you may want to ask:

- How long is the track to partnership?
  - What does that track involve?
- Is there a hard asset and/or AR buy-in or simply a par value for stock (eg, 1 share of stock = $10,000)
- How many MDs have been hired in the last 5 years?
  - Of those MDs, how many are still with the group?
- Is there a buy-in/buy-out?
  - If so, what are the details?

Other questions might include asking whether anyone has previously **not** been offered partnership who was on a partnership track. That could be a sign as to the stability of the group. How many MDs have they turned over in the last 5 years? A high number is definitely a sign of something gone afoul. Have MDs left the group voluntarily? Ditto. And, your goal is to become a partner. But what *if* you elect NOT to become a partner? Are you allowed to simply stay as an employed physician? (Generally not in your best interest, from a career perspective.) This is all about balance. It's about balancing professional demands with personal needs, about balancing interest in the practice with obsession, and about finding a cohesive fit that enables you to grow professionally and personally.

If you've gotten a good handle on the group and its cohesion, in my humble opinion, you've obtained a grasp for what your experience might be like in the future. If these guys get along, the more the merrier. If they do not, that could portend trouble.

## THE NUMBERS – YOUR CONTRACT AND FUTURE BUY-IN/BUY-OUT

This is not my forte, but I can speak to some of the particulars of employed-physician contracts. Remember, almost anything is negotiable. If a car dealer wants to move a car, he'll deal. If a furniture salesman is dying to make way for the newest line, she'll deal. If a practice really needs you, they'll deal. I know you have more training and intellectual capital, and comparing you to wheeler-dealers is inappropriate, but you get the point.

When you've made it this far, and you've decided this is the right fit, you should understand some basics about the contract with which you're about to be presented.

Here are some keys to be privy to:

1. Contracts normally run for an initial term of 1 year, and they'll generally run with the same terms until you're at the threshold of partnership. So, it could be for 1 year or 5 years, depending on when partnership hits. The initial couple of paragraphs will likely speak to your exclusive work with the practice, unless you receive written authorization to go outside of your duties, a word or two about proper notice of intent to terminate, etc.

2. Compensation will normally be delineated in a paragraph. Make sure that you understand the language, especially if there are bonuses or other distributions involved in your compensation. If the formula to calculate a bonus is complicated, putting it in writing and understanding it as you read it can be challenging. My suggestion with compensation is to ask for it to be delineated in simple numbers so you can at least, in theory, understand how the calculations work and how the dollars might flow to you. This assures that there are no misunderstandings.

3. There may be a paragraph discussing your duties for the business, where and when you're expected to work (eg, in the state of Mississippi) and offering which/what types of medical services.

4. There will be a discussion about your vacation, meetings, and CME travel, and the related costs and allowances, on an annual basis.

5. There will be a handful of paragraphs full of boilerplate legalese that have meaning to attorneys and their ilk. (Eg, what defines this, what defines that, etc.)

6. There will be something tucked into the contract regarding non-competes. Just so you know, many courts (this is anecdotal) have not recognized non-competes, because in some areas of the country it's been deemed that there is a need for the MD's specialty (eg, an underserved area). The courts have recognized the community's health care needs over the needs of the practice. However, even if a non-compete could be invalidated by the court, many times there are compensation

components woven into the non-compete in the event that the non-compete does not hold. There would be a fairly robust cash outlay due from you to the practice immediately upon terminating your contract to protect the practice from the downside of an unenforceable non-compete, should you decide to see patients in the practice's current geographic or service area. A non-compete should also be well defined and reasonable.

7. Paragraphs speaking to med/mal insurance you must carry (due to a corporate decision) are usually $1,000,000/$3,000,000, meaning you're covered for $1 million per occurrence and $3 million in aggregate should you be hit with a med/mal suit. Discussion will also address the prospect of tail coverage (prior acts) if the practice is on a claims made policy vs an occurrence policy. Ask the group what their med/mal insurance is, claims made or occurrence. Most groups will not pay your tail coverage from your prior employer but they may, depending on their situation, be willing to split the cost or work out some other arrangement. Remember, these points *may* be negotiable.

8. A paragraph will cover reimbursable business expenses and the like.

9. Another paragraph will discuss, very specifically, termination with and without cause and what conspires to make either, such as loss or forfeiture of medical license, abuse of controlled substances, etc. Make sure that with/without cause is defined very clearly so that nebulous definitions open to interpretation are not included in your contract.

10. There'll be discussion of disability pay and what qualifies an MD as disabled.

11. A paragraph may be included dealing with discussion on the medical records and who owns them (usually the practice).

The aforementioned was a non-exhaustive list. These are some basics you might look for in your contract. When you've found that magical, nirvana-esque position, you should work a little to negotiate components of the employment agreement that you'd like, knowing there may be push back and knowing, once again, what your balance is. What can you live with and live without? You might also ask whether or not all contracts are uniform.

In terms of negotiating your contract, remember there are a couple of points, at least as you are looking for employment, which may be malleable and open to discussion. They include:

a. If the contract contains salary guarantees with financial assistance provided by a local/area hospital, the agreements can get complicated but the onus, generally, falls on you and the hospital. Those agreements can no longer be between the hospital and the practice you'll work for, due to the government's concerns regarding kick-backs and the like.

b. There may be an opportunity for some student loan forgiveness.

c. There may be the opportunity for a one-time sign-on bonus.

d. Maybe the group will offer you and your family health and dental insurance.

e. There may be a dollar allocation for moving expenses if you need to relocate to take the position.

## THE BUY-IN

After the employment period, in most cases you'll be offered the option to buy into partnership. It is worthwhile, after interviewing and moving the process forward, to contemplate the buy-in/buy-out entailed in partnership. You want as much information as possible *before* you sign your *employment* contract, which means you need to know what the future may hold in store for you after the term of your employment has run its course and you are preparing to buy in to the business.

The reason for this is your buy-in path may equate to upwards of a 2-year hitch as an employee. You would hate more than anything to be in a job you love, in an area you adore, with a quality of life you've heretofore dreamed about, to find out, when the partnership documents arrive, that you are basically an indentured servant for the next 5 years while you work off your buy-in or work into an equity position within the practice. Could you elect to overlook some of this, you know, because you love the job? Entirely so. But why would you? This is an area where you need to look out for number 1, no matter how collegial the group. Ultimately, there is the possibility that on your way to buy in you get slugged with some surprises that make you very unsettled, that fracture the fragile shell of comfort you've established with your employers and soon-to-be partners.

Remember, if it's not in writing, your agreement is predicated on recollection and memory, which oftentimes is open to interpretation and can be hampered by convenient amnesia. Having opined that, once you have an offer on the table and your foot in the door, I'd ask to see the partnership agreements and documents. I'd obtain the buy-in information when you're near a deal. Promises that "we'll take care of you" are cozy, neat, and make a guy feel loved, but those promises become malleable when stretched over the employment period. Many of the promises and their value depends on who in the practice you've talked to, who in the group is pulling the strings, and who, ultimately, has the authority. These warm fuzzies are probably rendered from the heart, but when push comes to shove, you have no one to fall back on but yourself, and hollow commitments of "love" will quickly leave you heartbroken on the shoals of disenchantment in the years following your employment. Remember, people—especially busy people—have very short memories. Getting things down in writing can be invaluable.

If the group will not offer the partner documents, an alternative might be for a senior MD, the Managing Partner, or even the administrator to give you a very simple example of how the buy-in works, in easy-to-use round numbers with no sharp edges (eg, in terms used in this book: $100 to buy 10 shares of stock, etc) so that you can draw some conclusions of your own, to craft better and more salient questions to ask your impending employer. Even round, soft numbers can give you an idea of how the process works, and that is most of what you want to know. Practices should not hide the calculations of the buy-in formula from you unless they have something to hide.

Once you have some basic numbers, sit with your accountant and/or an experienced advisor. Don't slough this stuff off on your neighbor Fred who's "good with agreements" or equally "good with numbers." Health care management is not rocket science, but conversely, rocket science is not health care management. Each requires its own set of disciplines and attention to detail. An experienced advisor can offer you insight into the agreement, can compare its demands and peculiarities with those of other agreements s/he has seen in the past, and offer you comprehensive counsel. While some agreements may not offer you much wiggle room on the language ("This is the contract we've used forever") it will at least give you a heads up on some of the pitfalls you're about to head into. At least knowing how deep the water is prior to jumping in will lend some comfort to the prospect of landing. Quite frankly, if the group you're courting loves you that much, they should be willing to offer reasonable concessions in the agreement, to undergo a little give and take, if you will.

Occasionally you'll hear "we don't change our buy-in for anyone." That may or may not be true. There can come a time when the need for a new subspecialty (eg, EP vs a general cardiovascular MD) necessitates some flexibility on the negotiating side regarding the contract. Say, hypothetically, that the practice's last MD hire was 10 years ago. Now suppose that, due to growth in the tiny community, the group finds itself with the need to add 2 more MDs. They go out expecting to pay $100,000/year plus med/mal, maybe some life insurance, 3 weeks of vacation, and a 3-year track to *buy-in*. They run an ad with their local and national specialty associations and receive very impressive CVs. When they begin the interview process, they learn at the outset that the new crop of MDs want $250K, a sign-on bonus, 5 weeks off (including 1 week of CME), and partnership in 2 years. What to do? Well, if all MD candidates seem in line with these demands, the practice may need to ponder working with the selected candidate and get the deal done. There are myriad numbers of ways with which to bring all to the table and make a fit.

Performing this legwork, painful and slow though it is, may save you considerable heartburn when you're getting ready to pull the trigger with your partners.

As an aside, your employment contract is just that. It is exclusive of partnership commitments or offers. In fact, some contracts actually say that the owners will review the employed physician's prospect of partnership when the time comes. As you can see, just as with life, there are no guarantees with contracts, so be sure to examine the language in your contract relative to a potential future offer of partnership.

Oftentimes, the buy-in is constructed of a variety of components. Many agreements have boilerplate language that is fairly basic and somewhat similar to an employment contract, involving such things as non-competes, delineation of assorted agreed-upon benefits, your commitment to work only for the group while you're employed, etc. The key aspects to the partnership agreement lie in the dollars and cents of the buy-in and its timeframe. These take a variety of forms, shapes, and sizes, and this is not the venue to delve into each in depth. Outside of the general language in the contract, a non-exhaustive list of possible components incorporated into a buy-in includes:

1. **Goodwill** – generally an intangible derived from a perceived value of the practice based on its history in the area; basically, how long it has built a reputation and standing in the community. Some practices, dare I say, have managed to generate "negative" goodwill by acting like, well, jerks to area referrals, clinicians, and patients. Regardless of the mathematical machinations involved, this measure becomes fairly subjective in nature. I would also inquire as to whether or not the goodwill number includes the purchase of any other practice in the past.

   a. Sometimes practices purchase other practices and their goodwill. This can involve purchasing of depreciated hard assets, too. If charts are purchased from other practices, a dollar value is attributed to this transaction. Just so you know, as far as I'm concerned charts have a value, on an ongoing basis, of between $0 and $0 x 1 (translation: worth nothing). Why? Quite simply it's because you can't buy a chart. Look at it pragmatically. Let's say Fred X, MD, has 10,000 charts in his vast collection accumulated over 20 years in practice. Good Dr X has decided he's tired for working hard, 80 hours a week, and making less than he did in the early 1980s. Dr X brings in consultant Y to help him value the charts. In theory, what you'd be looking for is some innate value in continued patient visits, generally based on patient history or medical condition. This might translate into future revenue streams. But how can you be assured of continued access to this patient population? You can't. Remember, patients vote with their feet. If you, as the new kid on the block, are not liked by the patients Dr X had, for whatever reason, they can leave. If you've paid $10,000 for their charts, a mere $1/chart, you are now out some piece of $10,000, depending on how many folks remain with you. Not a good buy. Sometimes these deals are thrown in to practice purchases.

Anyhow, I hope you see where I'm coming from. In buying a practice, *almost* NO argument can be made for purchasing charts of patients. Again, patients are under no obligation to see you and there are no guarantees.

2. **Hard assets** (equipment and the like) – generally some depreciated value of an asset or assets is included in a buy-in. The reason for this is that the assets have a value on the balance sheet and can fairly easily be quantified. The depreciated value of the asset is delineated as such. If the practice purchased a $1,000,000 Ooogaflagmobomitor 3 years ago, using straight-line depreciation for 5 years (the asset depreciates in equal amounts over the Oooga's useful life) would mean that the Oooga is now worth, as a depreciated asset, $400,000. $1,000,000/5 years of depreciable life = $200,000/year in depreciation. Three years of depreciation is $200,000 x 3 = $600,000. So the Oooga would be valued at somewhere around a $400,000 asset on the books of the practice, and shows that the practice has assets worth at least $400,000, something tangible to buy into.

3. **Accounts Receivable** (AR) – AR are the outstanding revenues, or accounts receivable, that the practice has on the books for charges out to Medicare, private-pay insurance companies (eg, BC/BS, UnitedHealthcare, etc), and patients. Accounts receivable, in a normal business model, would be the money we are waiting to be paid by our business clients. They owe us for performing services. The same holds true for health care.

When looking at this component, make certain that AR, when included in a buy-in calculation, is reduced to a collectible amount. While in normal business we might expect to collect *everything* we bill, health care is not that animal. Instead, you'll expect to collect a percentage of what you've billed. That is to say, the practice will not collect its entire AR. You'll get a better understanding of AR later in the book. Most importantly, you should ask the practice you are courting what their collection percent of collectible money is and what percent they collect on their accounts receivable. While you're at it, ask them what their AR value is. More than informative for you, this can serve as a test for a practice manager or senior partner. A practice with good management and a good handle on their dollars outstanding should be able to reel this figure off with little or no problem. AR can be a component of the buy-in process, so understanding what AR means is essential to you.

Aside from the dollars and cents, let's say you have a 3-year buy-in track, maybe a fixed salary that creeps up incrementally after each year of employment, and then the big watershed moment; you buy-in. What else are you buying into, exactly? What's your role in the group? Do you want a more active or passive role in the day-to-day decision-making processes? Are you paying into a pyramid scheme, the results of which amount to you propping up unproductive senior docs who begin phasing out their effort but not tweaking back their pay commensurate with their workload reduction?

(Eg, a reduction in call or reduction in office hours.) If there are 10 partners in the group, where do you fall? Is there a seniority ranking? Or are you just becoming a partner and paying a premium to have no voice and no vote? This is where structure may be important to you. You'd want to know that your voice has some value to the organization, either on a standing or ad hoc committee or some other avenue. (Like a budget finance committee or a marketing committee or physician disciplinary committee [did I just type that??].)

Make sure, when all is said and done, that you have a qualified attorney review your contract. The money invested in this process can protect you and offers you peace of mind.

## REFERENCES

1. http://www.cbsnews.com/stories/2006/08/29/health/main1948318.shtml
2. http://aspe.os.dhhs.gov/progsys/forum/issform.htm
3. http://aspe.os.dhhs.gov/progsys/forum/issform.htm
4. http://aspe.os.dhhs.gov/progsys/forum/issform.htm
5. http://aspe.os.dhhs.gov/progsys/forum/issform.htm
6. *MGMA Connexion,* August 2007, pp. 20&21
7. *ibid*
8. *ibid*
9. http://www.piedmonthealthcare.com/piedmont/index.asp
10. http://www.amga.org/WhoWeAre/index_whoWeAre.asp
11. http://www.trailblazerhealth.com/Tools/Fee%20Schedule/MedicareFeeSchedule.aspx
12. http://www.trailblazerhealth.com/Tools/Fee%20Schedule/MedicareFeeSchedule.aspx

# BOOK TWO

# *On To Business*

## THE NUTS AND BOLTS OF
## THE PRIVATE PRACTICE

AS A GENTLE REMINDER, this is no all-inclusive book. Remember, our goal here is to broadly enlighten, educate, and hopefully make you smile a few times whilst offering the aforementioned components. It would be a disservice for me to try to tell you that you could boil down such a truly complicated model into a 150 or so page book. We want to cover as much ground as possible so that you can get a good feel for what to expect and what to look for in a limited amount of space.

When you head into a practice you're interested in, you should, just by looking around, be able to garner an understanding about its infrastructure. In this case, I mean medical equipment (nuclear cameras, echo machines, imaging modalities) and management. It is telling if all of their equipment was skillfully handcrafted before the incandescent light bulb came into existence or was newer, say, when the long playing (LP) album came into being. Also, if they have only one manager trying to handle a 10-doc group with 65 employees, they're decidedly short on management infrastructure. Shortchanging the practice's needed infrastructure and capital investments can be a big mistake.

It's important to store in the back of your mind as you move along in this process that you're getting ready to enter a business. I know I've said it before and I just might keep saying it lest we forget: This is a business, just like Coke or McDonald's, but on a smaller scale. You will now be in the realm of a *very* regulated industry, with laws established by the federal government designed, essentially, to assure that MDs are not seeing and referring patients to entities who offer them money for that pleasure: rules that govern physicians' rights to own certain entities in health care in which they might have a financial relationship via ownership. You are moving into a very sticky zone.

To add to that excitement, though, you have the business components of your . . . business. That is to say, while you're busy trying to juggle and understand Stark laws, you must also be cognizant of *normal* small business concerns, such as the business's exposure to sexual harassment, all the rules and regulations that guide minimum wage, the myriad laws regarding 401K and profit-sharing plans, hiring/firing rules under the Equal Employment Opportunity Commission (EEOC), the Health Insurance Portability and Accountability Act (HIPAA), and all the other fun stuff inherent therein. You are preparing to enter a business, odd though the business model may be, and you need to begin thinking like a business owner. So, in short, not only are you concerned with providing the best medicine you can in a conscientious, efficient manner, but you're concerned that your partners are not sexually harassing anyone or firing anyone without due process.

One thing to remember, and we'll hit this point again and again, is as with a marriage, people do not change. And you won't change the MDs in the group. If you've got a bad vibe about a practice, don't think you're going to go in there and save everyone's soul. It won't happen. I've seen plenty of gung-ho MDs fire into a practice, bound and determined to make changes, to show the senior guys all the benefits of youth and vitality, only to slowly but surely (and inexorably) transform into the prototypical sample of the long-time physicians on hand at the practice, their hopes and dreams dashed against the rocks of internal intransigence and institutional inertia. See, at some point the new MD sees that s/he can only beat his/her head against the wall for so long before they're made aware of 2 sobering realities. Those are, in no particular order, that the wall won't move and that their head will bleed.

When looking at a private medical practice, I believe that one of the qualities ultimately defining the success of the group is physician involvement. You should inquire about physician input and interest in the numbers and monthly reports, staff evaluations, and the like. This keen interest in the group's soft, white underbelly should go some way in letting you know how involved the MDs are in making things run and, by extension, how much they *truly* know about their practice and what makes it tick.

MDs don't, and shouldn't, need to know when staff comes in, clocks out for lunch, and leaves for the day, unless that staff member impacts that MD's clinical day. Otherwise, leave the ultimate day-to-day details to qualified management. No, when I speak to MD involvement in the group, I'm talking about the MD's knowledge and exposure to their group. Do they know what their overhead is? Does the manager know the basic tenet of "profit?" That is, total revenue - total cost = profit. Heck, do they know what the *term* "overhead" is? Do they know how many staff members they have? How many full-time equivalents (FTEs) they have? Not all of these are fatal to miss. For instance, more than likely 70%-80% of MDs do not know how many FTEs they actually have. They should know, though, how their group functions. Because, from a management perspective, there's nothing more frustrating than taking orders from a boss who has no idea what s/he is talking about.

Micro-managing MDs bring no value to the group. That much I know with certainty. They clog the works and slow people down, often times asking multiple people to accomplish the same task, changing the task multiple times in a limited time period (say a week), asking that energy be spent on a non-mission critical adventure, and generally trying to be hands-on when the situation dictates hands-off. (Recall, it's all about balance.)

On the flip side, MDs who are passive about their group, about the impact of outside forces (payers, both private [BC/BS, for instance] and public [read Medicare/Medicaid]), and their competitive stance relative to their community peers, are soon to be run over. There is no longer any room out there for the passive clinician. There will come a time, if your employment involves a partnership track, when you'll begin the buy-in process in the years to come; you're making an investment in your future business and the people across the table from you are soon to be your business partners, warts and all.

That said, the organization of the group you're looking to join is tantamount to your growth as a practitioner, your stability, and your longevity in your chosen geographic area. There are few things more damaging to the success of a medical practice than over-inflated egos coupled with a lack of interest in a group experience, topped off with a smattering of bad personality fits. I've seen it before. And it's a mess. Although emotionally dysfunctional groups can survive, I'd suggest to you that they cannot thrive, and the hidden turmoil that tickles the surface inevitably seeps into the very fiber of the group, leaches into the group's very culture, and does untold damage.

## *Group Structure—Non-tax related*

When I speak to structure, I think of it in essentially 2 ways. The first was mentioned above in Book One. It entailed a practice's structure, for tax purposes. The second is the organizational structure. I contemplate the organization of the group itself. That is, who's in charge? Who reports to whom? Those answers are helpful, as they'll offer you a better understanding of where you might fit in the pecking order. If you're looking at a medium-sized group (say 5-10 physicians), it might be helpful to know who the managing partner is, so that when you interview, you can get a vibe from him or her as to how they interact, how they treat you: the newbie. Structure is important to understand, as it poses how the clinicians mesh apropos of the business parameters.

How is the group put together? Do they have a domineering senior doc who thinks (or acts) like his opinion is *the* one that matters? This type of structure is unhealthy for the organization. There are also practitioners out there who want to manage the practice, as the managing partner or CEO, and want to maintain an MD's salary. This is untenable and unrealistic. Generally the business cannot afford, nor should it attempt, to pay a physician who is neither seeing patients nor generating a revenue of $200,000-$400,000 a year to manage the practice. That's what people like me are for. Managerial talent is out there if you look, it'll cost a fraction of an MD's salary, and that talent will most probably know more about running an organization than an MD will.

## FUN/EDUCATIONAL ANECDOTE NUMBER 3

I know you're not laughing at me regarding the managing partner making more than $200,000 to run the practice full time. I know that you think the aforementioned salary is an overstated absurdity to prove the absurd, an outlandish claim to back an argument, right? Let me tell you that I was privy to someone in that situation not too long ago, and the MD salary in question was *more than* the high end on the continuum mentioned above.

Anyhow, back to my point about structure. The question evolves to: "Is all of the power of decision making in the group vested in one person?" And if that's so, is that ok with you? Obviously, if you're joining a one-man/-woman group, this might be ok with you, as that "decider" is probably the guy/gal who founded the group and got the thing off the ground. One would hope that if you're in a small group, all hands can work together to steer the ship, coming to, where possible, consensus about all things practice-related. If not, do you want to invest your time in this situation? If you join a group, remember one very salient thing. There is a premium to joining a group. The reason for this is that your predecessors have dedicated long hours, blood, sweat, toil and, in many cases, family, to make this business run. Ponder this, if you would. Running a small business, no matter the business, can be very challenging. Try practicing medicine all day long and *then* running a business. Put another way, get into practice for a year or so. See how you feel after work. Then think about investing another 2-3 hours a night into the business side of the practice: your business. Only then will you appreciate what the guys/gals before you went through.

One thing is for certain. You don't want to be in a situation where your opinion, partner or not, does not matter. I've not seen many groups where the partners completely exclude the newbies from the important decisions. First, including you will work for the owners, because it provides evidence of your interest in the group, soon to be your part out of "X" owners. Additionally, it's a low-cost way of getting you involved in the group and at least seemingly offers you some input.

It works for you for the same reasons. Even if the ultimate decisions are not yours, it's nice to be included, even if it's just your perception. You never want a position where the senior physician has the *only* opinion that matters, thereby rendering the place a virtual dictatorship. It will work for no one and remember our mantra: you can't change the person you're marrying.

In larger groups, let us say 5 or more physicians, there should be a functioning Board with an executive committee. Normally, the Board is comprised of the shareholders, or partners. The executive committee is normally a small subset of the Board which, in theory, is nimble (due to its limited membership), allowing it to work with the practice management staff to quickly decide and effect the management-related work of the practice. If there's an executive committee subset, that group often has a reporting mechanism back to the greater board, thereby keeping them informed of the goings-on in the practice, imbued with a nominal spending authority (so that they don't slow down the process and progress by constantly running to the Board for approval of every pencil they want to purchase), and ostensibly assisting the Administrator in carrying out the will of the Board via the Executive Committee. Votes are normally either via a majority, super majority, or other vote that will carry forward, deliberately and thoughtfully, the wishes of the physician owners.

Fortunately, there's good news in a large group. (More lenient call schedules, market power in negotiating, etc.) But there's also a problem. When practices begin to get larger they also can get a bit more unwieldy. At that point, it is almost required that an executive committee be empowered to handle the managing of the business. There might even be a Managing Partner with the authority to make day-to-day decisions with the administrator. However, as the group grows, the opportunity to find consensus generally wanes proportionally. There's probably some sort of provable inverse relationship between the group's size and the actual involvement of all MDs, employed or owners. Keep in mind, as the group gets bigger, this nearly cries out for a formalized feedback loop so all Partners are looped into what transpires with the senior team and administration. Nothing rankles MDs more than being out of the loop.

## *What to Look For—Top Down*

### STRATEGIC PLANNING

What is the philosophy guiding the ship? What is their plan? Does the group you're interviewing have a strategic plan? If so, ask them for what duration of time. They may not be interested in letting you read the plan, obviously, as it would give away the keys to the castle. But they should be willing let you see that the document exists or you might ask them to elaborate on how your addition to the practice fits in with their overall vision. That'd throw them!

A strategic plan, by its nature, is fluid and dynamic, a living testament to the group's plan put on paper and memorialized. It is comprised of assumptions drawn in the present, based on current and recent historical data, and on fundamental decisions and actions seen right now as necessary to attain practice goals. The plan must be dynamic, given the health care climate, and the practice must have in place the infrastructure designed to react to those changes smoothly and quickly, adjusting both operations and the plan to meet the needs of the dynamic marketplace. A strategic plan is a document that delineates how the group will get to its vision. Normally crafted for up to 3 years, a strategic plan can have a horizon of 5 years. However, deviation from a plan that far out into the future grows exponentially the further you get away from Day 1 of implementation. I think this is particularly true most especially in health care, as the dynamic changes with frequency and flux.

To give the plan value, the physicians must recognize and fully embrace the defined objectives and resources and remain focused on both. The strategic plan should be reviewed annually, at a minimum, to see if the path the group is on, given the data available when the plan was drafted, is accurate and still validates the plan and its direction. The strategic plan is used to define and measure goals, but ultimately it will require constant attention where we evaluate the goals and revisit their wisdom in light of external influences.

## VISION AND MISSION STATEMENTS

The group's first strategic plan should have identified a vision and a mission statement. Some folks will poo-poo the vision and mission statements. That's fine, because many groups succeed and flourish quite well, thank you, without either of those 2 components. But what they provide is the result of introspection, of thought and deliberation by the partners, as to which way the group is headed. And this introspection translates into a workable plan for the management team and staff.

Even if a group does not at least have a mission or a vision defined on paper, that does not mean no planning is taking place. The group might have a semblance of a strategic plan, or even a fully fleshed out strategic plan.

*Vision*

Some groups, though I'd suggest to you not many, have a vision that they use as a touchstone for their future planning and a mile marker, if you will, towards actualizing the group's future. This exercise is more often than not stumbled through in a haphazard manner, where the vision happens more than is planned out. In other words, practices will head in the direction they think they need to go but don't do so, in many instances, consciously. A vision is best when it's pondered, defined, and contemplated in the scheme of the overall group. It requires very real thought and introspection because the vision is where you are trying to go. It offers the group an endpoint. For instance, if you're a 5-doc cardiology group in Hartford, Connecticut, might it be your vision to be a 10-MD group in 5 years, with physicians specializing in CT angiography? Would the group make the statement, as part of their vision, that they will ". . . offer cardiology services to areas north of I-84 and will be a full-service cardiovascular group"? This is a simple vision that delineates a geographic area in which the group intends to operate, a defined number of clinicians (hopefully based on some sound supply-and-demand figuring), and a finite timeframe in which it wants to reach this goal. All tied up in a nifty sentence. The vision can then be addressed and modified in annual strategic planning to see if, over the course of time, it'll pass the limits of the needs of the group.

*Mission Statement*

A mission statement gives vitality and life to the group's vision and direction. As with the vision, the mission requires contemplation and deliberation, taking stock and evaluating what the group is doing and why. The mission focuses on the *purpose* of the organization and the purpose of what the practice is in business to do. It should lend pithy affirmation to the definition of what the group hopes to achieve.

For instance, that same cardiology group in Hartford might have a mission of "...providing compassionate care to you and your loved ones and holding your cardiovascular health in as high esteem as you do." One note on the mission and other statements. I'd caution you from making quality statements that cannot be verified in something as nebulous as disease outcomes. Saying in your mission, for instance, that "we will provide you with the highest quality cardiovascular care imaginable" leaves you open to some potential downsides. What if Suzy Q's husband dies in your care? And what if she says ". . . you said you'd provide the highest quality care imaginable and you did not because Mr Q has died." Well, you're in a bit of a pickle, aren't you? I mean, you probably worked hard to save Mr Q, but did you really provide him with the "highest quality of care imaginable?" If you think so, how would you qualify, or quantify, that? In any event, that bold mission statement might be a touch overly ambitious and could be used against you in a court of law while you face a jury of your peers. You see where this is heading.

What a group's mission, vision, and strategic plans will show you is that the group actually took the time to envision their future, actually went through the exercise of pondering who they are and where they want to be. Though they may not follow it to a T, they sat down and planned for the growth of the practice.

You should keep in mind that strategic plans and business plans are different animals. A strategic plan, generally, is a brief description of the group's plan for the near future. A business plan is a very detailed document which includes a financial analysis, a business growth prospectus, etc, and is usually proffered as a precursor to the business, delineating very clearly what the business hopes to achieve, how it will be financed, and so on. Business plans are large documents created to offer insight into things like financing, analysis of customers, service base, etc.

Other innocuous, though useful, questions apropos of the strategic plan and overall vision include asking when the practice had its last planning meeting if they've hit, or are hitting, their targets and goals. After all, setting a plan without measurable outcomes is analogous to spitting into the wind, no?

## SUMMARY

The strategic plan, vision, mission, and components of the organization can be, on their face, fairly telling about how things are, or are not, run. A group that can whip out an organizational chart, delineate their vision, and discuss the status of their strategic plan is going in the right direction. This shows a certain attention to detail, attention paid to the pieces that make the thing work, and hopefully assures that the ups are high and the downs are mitigated in their severity. After all, you're getting ready to embark on a fairly wild ride. You don't want it to be too manic.

## THE ORG CHART

Organization charts are useful in graphically depicting who reports to whom and a logical flow of information. The boxes on these charts should have job descriptions that are associated with the jobs delineated in the boxes.

Exhibit 5 offers a sample org chart. This might be a chart deployed by one of the very large groups we mentioned earlier in the book. That is, the group that has somewhere north of 30 physicians (not including extenders such as PAs and nurse practitioners) reporting through the chain of command.

## MANAGING PARTNER

Normally, this is an MD who is empowered by the Board to handle, with the administrator, the day-to-day tasks of running the group, with weekly (or some other consistent mechanism) reports back to the physicians of the Board. The managing partner position is often a position voted on by the partners in the group with some sort of term-limited parameter. It's best to have someone who understands the business basics and who understands some, if not all, of the fundamentals inherent in running a practice. S/he should comprehend with a basic understanding business components, such as what overhead is and how that ratio is calculated, what the practice's comfort with their overhead rate is, and what general, basic, and capital equipment components cost. (eg, a new cardiovascular nuclear camera may run the practice between $200,000-$225,000.)

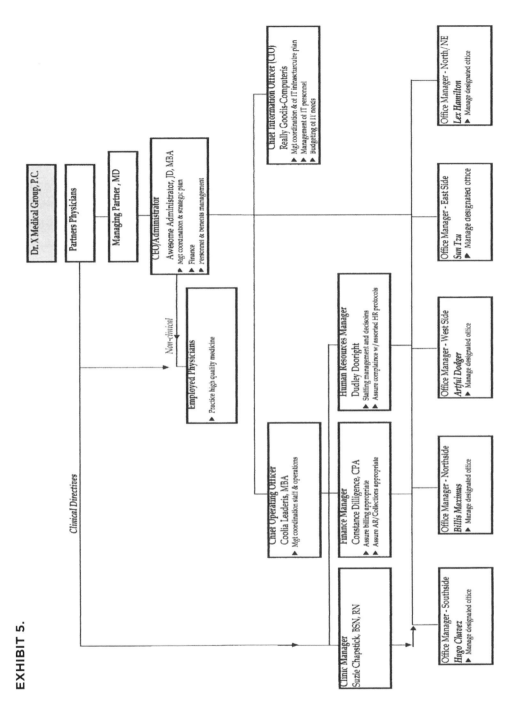

**EXHIBIT 5.**

A basic understanding makes it easier for the managing partner to work with the administrator, who is intimately involved with such concerns on a daily basis. What you don't want to run into is the managing partner who proffers this sage, yet tried and true paradigm apropos of the practice's finances and how Partners might earn more in a given year:

## FUN/EDUCATIONAL ANECDOTE NUMBER 4

"We need to see more patients and cut our costs." Just so you know:

1.  This ditty was actually relayed to me via an associate whose managing partner said this to him/her, and
2.  This is what a good administrator is watching on a daily basis.

The managing partner can be a double-edged sword and here's why: you want an MD who's plugged in, who, as we say, gets it, but you don't want one who is overly intrusive on an hourly or even day-to-day basis. That is confining, restricting, and unnecessarily ties management's hands, prohibiting them from doing what they're supposed to do. So again, finding balance between an inherent knowledge of the group and weighing that vs your need to understand the business is essential. Remember, you need to know your business, to understand the basics and building blocks. You don't need to run it. That's why you hire good, qualified staff. And if you try to run it on a day-to-day basis, that is, try to micro-manage it, you'll drive people insane, in absolute terms, and end up doing a fairly bad job while scaring off good staff.

At your visit, ask the Managing Partner or the Administrator if you might see a copy of their business's organization chart. This chart (exhibit 5) displays, graphically, who reports to whom and what that means to the organization. I'd also ask about the terms or duration of each of the offices held and ask the administrator and/or managing partner about the functionality of each office in addition to how it influences the business. For instance, the managing partner might be in that role for 3 years and then a vote taken by the Board might amend that. Remember, the managing partner (MP) is usually some sort of bridge between the management staff and the physician leadership. As such, he will *also* have a day job. To wit: seeing patients. MP is a pretty thankless job, from time to time, with little pay for the job and headaches commensurate with the practice's organization. Some MP positions receive a stipend in addition to their MD salary, or some additional days off in lieu of a stipend, or maybe both.

## STAFF

We've spent the first half of this book examining what you need to look for in a medical practice. My belief, after doing this job for so many years, is that this book can save even the most seasoned MD. Initially, I set out to build this manuscript for Fellows and Residents, but I then considered how many MDs in practice knew very little about the business of medicine or didn't want to spend the next 5 years trying to get their heads around the business side of medicine while they practiced medicine. It's a tough nut and, as you know, time is probably the most precious commodity you have.

Now, with this new and improved delivery method that you've wrapped your hands around and invested in, you too can get an education in medical practice management.

We're going to now dive headlong into the bread and butter of a medical practice organization. We're going to consider staff, the numbers, and some other odds and ends. It's my hope that this will give you a look under the hood, a look at what makes the thing run, a junior (and unaccredited) MBA with a concentration in health care.

The importance of good, highly trained staff cannot be measured. And yet, a medical group's management team must do just that. As I've said, I'm of the mind that you help good people to the next level, you give the mediocre performers a chance and the tools to do better, and you show the less qualified people out the door. It's that simple. You don't have time to try to keep all people happy all of the time. It's disingenuous and potentially harmful to the group. And one message on that. You need to stick by your management when they're right. You need to see both sides of the argument, just like you'd evaluate multiple treatment options for a disease state. But when all is said and done, you need to remove the emotion from the decision-making process. Let's say you have a nurse who's fun-loving and nice. But she thinks she's been touched by Midas. As such, she thinks she's above everyone, including your management staff, (and maybe a doc or 2 in the group). Just so you know, this is **never**, (did you see that?), **never** acceptable! If you take staff's side in an argument (when they're wrong) because you like them, you do an unbelievable disservice to *your* business and undermine the management team. It's short-sighted and ultimately detrimental to your business. Don't get me wrong. Staff is not always wrong and legitimate beefs should be aired, vetted, and dealt with. They should be heard in the right context, in the right venue, and not in front of other staff. Staff should never hear, nor see, a break down in MD commitment to the management team and a lack of respect by the management to the MDs. It's a 2-way street. And, it is hoped, both players (eg, MDs and management) are professionals.

There are some poor managers out there and they deserve to be kept in line and/or shown their way out the door. But if you have a good manager, if you have good management staff, then you need to do the right thing and stick by them.

## FUN/EDUCATIONAL ANECDOTE NUMBER 5

Many moons ago, I'd worked with a single-specialty group in a land far, far away. It was a time of giant beasts that roamed the earth, when thick gaseous clouds of sulfur gas blanketed the world and blocked out the sun, painting streaks of pink and deep orange hues across the setting sun.

One of my managers came to me to let me know that Suzie Q, RN, was getting a perk that no one else was getting. We'll call it fire. And other staff members, we'll call them "the tribe," knew this. I asked how this could be, given the shortage of fire in the camp. Manager 1, we'll call him Quirt, explained that Suzie Q was a favorite of the Senior

Partner, who we'll call Borg. Well, apparently, Suzie Q determined that since Borg loved her, her particular benefit would go on and on, *ad nauseum, ad infinitum, ad forever*. I explained to Quirt that this was wrong, we needed to keep fire distributed evenly. Quirt told Suzie Q, who, instead of pitching her discussion to me, the *de facto* leader of the tribe (an interesting thing, passive aggressiveness: it permeates medical groups, for some unknown reason), she went to Borg to lobby him. Oh, she didn't have enough fire at home, oh the little Quogs didn't have enough fire to play with, and so on. So, Borg came to me. He said, "Suit, why can't Suzie Q have decidedly more fire than all the other tribe members? She's been with us a long time, I love her and cannot function here without her." Now, picture this. A man who pays a significant slice of my salary, a man who's helping make the widgets, a man who founded the company, is telling me that he is unhappy that Suzie Q cannot benefit from the fire.

Now, parity is as important in medical practice management as it is in any business. One thing you find early on in this business is the dictum that no good deed goes unpunished. This truism will present itself within 6 months of starting a job in health care. So parity, among physicians, among staff members, among . . . janitors . . . is crucial. It is crucial on an MD level, because if the administrator assures parity among the MDs, then MDs will trust that the administrator is looking out for their *business* and not Dr X's personal interests; they know that the administrator will always do what's right for the business. If you try to assist one MD, and it's not in parity with the others, then you'll forever hear about it and all MDS will eventually divine that you are willing to bend the rules. Even the MD whom you've helped will feel this way. It's like being married but dating the secretary. You eventually dump your wife to marry the secretary. But will your new wife (old secretary) ever really trust you? I mean, after all, you left your wife for her and were willing to cheat on your spouse. You see where I'm going with this.

In any event, in the instant case, in a tight span of about 8 seconds, I thought about my meager severance package, my wife and kids, grabbed a handful of Y-chromosomal fortitude, and said to Borg, "Borg, if I let Suzie Q have more fire, everyone in the tribe will think she gets all the good perks. It'll create dissension, irritation, and could, conceivably, open us up for some sort of discrimination issues."

Borg pondered this for a moment and said, "Ok. That makes sense. You tell her."

The moral to the story is that Borg heard the facts, contemplated the facts, and stood by management, thereby making the right decision.

Now, if I'd told Borg that I just wanted to give Suzie Q a bunch of garbage for no reason, well then he would be in his position to tell me no. Again, management is not always right. But when they are not, you owe it to them, yourself, and your partners to deal with them discreetly and in a manner that does not undermine their authority. After all, we're all human and we all, even MDs, make mistakes.

Your staff is one of the most expensive assets you have. You pour money and time into finding them, screening them, and training them. Hours and thousands of dollars go into grooming good employees. That's why I make the argument that you must try to work with those who are on the fence. Managers should be introspective when dealing with staff to determine if staff has received appropriate training, appropriate tools, and appropriate feedback. If you've provided them all of the tools they need and they cannot live up to the practice's expectations, then you need to cut your losses.

Now, treating staff well does not mean giving them everything that they want. The phrase *letting the inmates run the asylum* seems to come to mind. No, treating staff right means treating them as you'd like to be treated: courteously, with respect, and with the occasional "thank you." Kudos may be your least expensive way of showing your gratitude. Raises are good and raises are nice, but it has been shown that over time incremental raises have a diminishing return and that employees attain more satisfaction out of kudos and a good working environment.

As a manager, it's my job, in my opinion, to help people on to the next level. If, after a time, I do not have a job that fits their skill sets, then it might just be time for them to move on. That's the simple calculus in employee management. In theory, a good manager should groom employees to take over his or her job.

You may get to a point where a staff member has outgrown his job and may not have more room to grow within the group, thereby necessitating a new position elsewhere. At that point, what I do, if we cannot come to some agreement, is wish them well and tell them I wish we could've kept them.

The practices you are interviewing with should have an internal or external human resources person who helps management, and by extension the owners, place a value and worth on each job in the practice. Setting up accurate job descriptions and salary ranges based on data can go a long way to getting you there. For instance, in your new group you may pay a good RN between $50,000-$75,000 per year, depending on her duties and scope of responsibility. If the RN is looking for $80,000, two things can happen. You tell her no way, the position is not worth $80K. Or, you evaluate your current salary structure and determine that in your market you're underpaying your staff, or that position, and you elect to make some market-related adjustments. Before doing so, make sure you've done your homework. My suggestion is that you be on the north side of median compensation for all of your positions. You then make sure your benefits are solid. Then, you can leverage discussions with employees, stating that you feel your salaries are fair and your benefits package is exceptional.

Health care can be a high turnover industry. But the last 2 years that I was with a certain private practice, we had annual employee turnover in the 2%-5% range. Not bad, considering some groups will run 10%-20% turnover a year. Think about the knowledge that escapes your practice each time you replace a body. Ponder the pain you will have when trained bodies depart, leaving you with untrained staff. Before you experience this, let me tell you: it is painful for administration as well as physicians. If you have a mass exodus, think about all of the knowledge you'll need to impart to the newbies.

Feel free to ask your pending group what their turnover is, on an annual basis. I bet you may get a funny look and some "ers" and "ummms." Groups should have a feel for this number. It displays how in touch they are with the group's goings-on. Even if their annual turnover rate is 10%-20%, they should be able to explain the rate, delineate the market factors at work that substantiate the turnover rate, and explain how they're dealing with the high turnover. Keep it in mind. Because high turnover means you get a staff that's green. A staff that's green means that the physicians are going to do a lot of the grunt work because the old staff took with them the knowledge and the new staff is too new to be of any value.

So, a practice should have an idea of a position's worth. That is, an ophthalmic tech right out of high school with no practical experience in a private medical facility might get paid $14/hour (nearly what you were paid in Fellowship ☺). That equates, without benefits and taxes and all of the other gobbledygook that's thrown in there, to approximately $29,000 per year. Is $14/hour a good wage for a tech with no formal training or education? What I do know is that you need an idea of what the *market* will bear for that tech. If it'll bear $28/hour, well, then you are grossly underpaying your staff member and will need to make a decision that you are ok with this, and if s/he learns of the jobs paying $28/hour, you'll either need to adjust accordingly or just have the revolving door of techs. It's your decision. You need to know what you pay folks relative to your in-town competition. If that tech is good, nay, great, and s/he comes to you saying that s/he was just offered $19/hour at Drs Fred and Ted right down the street, the practice must decide whether or not it's worth it to give Tech X what amounts to more than a $10,000 raise when she, ostensibly, will continue to perform the same job for you as s/he has in the past. Doesn't make sense, does it?

Along those lines, never give staff the same raise to be equitable. Just so you know, raises, generally, should be merit-based, meaning Suzy Q has earned her raise. If you give Suzy Q a 3% raise, and Johnny Joe, an employee who is marginal at best, a 3% raise, what message(s) are you sending? I'll give you a second to ponder this, because for me this is intuitive. For you, maybe not so much, as yet. Ok, time's up. The message you give Suzy Q is "You're doing a great job and you've earned a 3% merit raise." What you've told Mr Joe (who knows in his heart of hearts that he's not worth a thing) that doing just about nothing earns you a raise, you reward mediocrity (him) and penalize quality (her). Now, you could say that no one will know what raise anyone else has received. Believe me, word about raises and benefits gets out, even when *verboten*. And I know that 3% of Suzy's salary (in a raise) may not translate, in dollars, to 3% of Johnny's, but they know they had received the same percentage. For many folks, that would be enough to get the ship rocking.

Good staff members are nearly as important to the organization as are good MDs. Sound silly? Sure it does. Right up until the point where you're asking a tech to get a 23-gauge needle and they offer you a set of forceps. Or you've asked the billing staff to keep an eye on your accounts receivable and you find they're busier keeping an eye on YouTube. Maybe you've spent months training that billing person on your computer system with all the bells and whistles and s/he decides to leave for a job across town and another $.25/hour; it happens.

As stated previously, there's a fine balance in the private practice of medicine. The balance of paying good staff good wages and offering them incentives and motivation to be more, and become what they can in the specialty in which they work, while maintaining an eye on the costs of your employees. Regardless of your specialty, employee costs are going to be one of your largest fixed expenses (fixed meaning they are there, regardless of how much money you generate) ranging from 19%-30% of your total revenue for the business. We'll go into that later in the book. Think of it in these terms. For every dollar you bring in to the practice in revenue, 19-30 cents goes to paying for employees and benefits. So, an argument can easily be made that it makes sense to keep employees happy and well trained so that they feel the love, they feel appreciated and needed vs feeling like a commodity there to be berated by the nearest MD in the office.

You can value employees, and show that you value employees, not only by salary increases but in letting them know what type of job you think they're doing. A kind word, the understanding of their efforts and what it takes to do the job, are priceless. Keeping staff happy can also mitigate medical malpractice claims and *qui tam* lawsuits. *Qui tam* is derived from the Latin saying, "*Qui tam pro domino rege quam pro se ipso in hoc parte sequitur*," which means, essentially, "He who sues for the king as well as for himself."[1] In other words, a disgruntled staff member can begin a suit on behalf of the government and be a party to that suit, ending up with a percentage of the settlement.

An FTE employee, whether an MD or a staff member, is expressed as the value of the number of hours worked by the employee. If you have a staff member who works 20 hours a week, that translates into about 1040 hours a year (20 hours x 52 weeks/year). If you have a staff member who works 10 hours each week, you're at about 520 hours worked per year. So, if you looked at these 2 people as your FTE employees, you'd note that you have .75 FTEs or three-fourths of a full-time person. A full-time person is usually measured in 2,080 hours worked in a year. So, the 2 folks above coupled with 4 full-time people (working 40 hours per week) would translate into 4.75 FTEs.

Before we leave the macro (overall) organization and the physician-drivers to look at the micro (detail), let's look at some staffing stats provided by the MGMA. "What is the average turnover rate for staff in medical practices?

The MGMA report *Performance and Practices of Successful Medical Groups* tracks turnover percentages for various positions in group practices. The medians for better performing practices in the 2008 report, with 2007 data are:

Receptionists and medical records staff....................................25.7%

Nursing and clinical support staff.............................................18.8%

Billing/collections and data entry staff.......................................8.6%

Courtesy of the MGMA.[2]

## TAKE A BREATHER AND RECONCILE

I hope you're seeing the logical transition to the exercise we're currently engaged in. You're about halfway through this book. There's much more to come. In sum, we've talked about what you're looking for, where you're looking to be, and what type of group you want to be in.

We then discussed what you might look for in salary and compensation, and then touched on some of the economic parameters that will temper lofty goals with reality. We then looked at group types and sizes. Finally, we touched down a bit on the MD side of the management structure equation. Now, we'll dig a bit deeper into the office management side before burrowing into some of the micro, that is, minute, day-to-day stuff that I neither expect you to fully understand nor gain a proficiency in. But it helps for you to know about it.

Too often is the time, even against my better counsel, that I've seen young MDs not only become partner but "become partner." What, you ask, are you talking about? Here's what I'm talking about. The young MD who comes in fired up, ready to make a difference in health care and the practice. He has energy, he's no longer someone's workhorse, and he wants to change things. He's on a 2-year partnership track. He puts in his time as an employee, works hard, and staff loves him. Then he starts his buy-in to partnership and the wheels begin to fall off. He takes on an air of superiority with the staff, who just a year or so ago he was cordial with and seemingly cared about. He begins to morph into this unseemly beast, this . . . Partner. And now he's one of them, sold his soul to the dark side. A Partner, with all the baggage and trappings that go along with the title. Yet again, the staff has lost another potential MD to the sins of Partnership.

Funny? Yup. Sad? Definitely. True story? You betcha. It happens all the time. I know that some of you out there will swear to me that this could never happen to you, but I'm sure that a fair percent of you, maybe as high as 70%-80%, will fall into this black hole, never to be salvaged again, a mere wisp of what you once were (and believed in) early in your 20s. Mark my words and keep it in mind. The symptom is the metamorphosis, but clinically presents as narcissism. Boil it down that even though you contract the psychological state, and even if you think you have it, you'll never admit it. Those around you won't bother to tell you out of love, respect, or apathy.

## FUN/EDUCATIONAL ANECDOTE NUMBER 6

Just so you know, I have seen this happen. And I've seen it more than once. I'll give you an example. In the recent past, as I was transitioning to a new position in a new state, I cautioned a young MD I had recently hired not to become a Partner. He knew exactly what I was talking about. He knew I was not dissuading him from buying in when the time came. We were on the same page, and for some time he assured me, over a couple of scotches, that he would not become Partner. He swore that he'd always hold the staff in high esteem, that he valued their opinions, and would always listen to and be there for them. Not 2 years later, as he ramped up to partnership, his commitments to the sanctity of those words quickly gave way to the dark side of partnership.

## FUN/EDUCATIONAL ANECDOTE NUMBER 7

Another example I've heard is the newbie who was employed in a large group and then, upon making partnership, strolled into the administrator's office and announced to him something to the effect of " . . . now that I'm a partner, you'll need to come to me with issues." To which the administrator rightfully responded that there was a reason for the physician Board and that was who he'd go to. He then thanked the young MD to alight from his office.

Look, I know you're busy. You have a hard job and it will only get more difficult. That much is true. With patients getting more educated regarding their conditions, and with the conspiracy of obesity running rampant in our consumption lifestyle in the US and its concomitant issues, it's tough to be an MD. I fully appreciate that. But also, your staff is the group that's there for you, the group that will look out for you if you throw them a few scraps, and I cannot emphasize enough how important I personally think it is that you be privy to staff concerns and work with those who work hard for you and get rid of those who do not. Reward the good, give tools to the marginal, and, if the marginal don't step up, move them out the door. Think of this as a group working toward the same mission. This symbiosis is essential in the efficient and effective operation of a medical business. I've seen many practices succeed, and fail, in regard to these key ingredients. You should know that, like most things, this relationship lives and breathes at the pleasure of the physician-owners of the medical group. Their interest or intransigence sets the table for the climate of the practice and, ultimately, its staff. That is why earlier I pointed out the need for physicians to have some involvement in the practice. After all, if they do not, why would staff? These folks dictate the culture of the organization. And once that culture is established, it's the dickens to change.

Remember our first graph on page 2, Decision Pyramid? With all of the variables, what you elect to do is predicated on your basic needs, wants, and desires. It's predicated on what blend of variables will actually make you happy with your choice and selection: MD involvement in the group, a cohesive mission, and talented individuals in place.

## MANAGEMENT STRUCTURE

As with the MDs, it's important to know, in terms of staff, who reports to whom. This is good for you and the staff. A well-defined organization chart, as mentioned previously, of staff and their jobs coupled with well-defined job descriptions will help you understand who you need to go to for various leadership, and assists staff in terms of reporting and who they're expected to please in the pecking order. One *faux pas* made by MDs is they often choose the path of least resistance to get things done and they will go to a staff member to do something when they should've gone to the manager or the administrator. What's the problem with this, you say? Aside from basically obviating the organization's hierarchy, it can give staff a mixed message, a mixed direction, on what they're supposed to be doing. It can also cause tremendous inefficiency and duplication of effort. It's generally a bad idea. Ostensibly, if the MD management team has decided on something, staff marching orders should be divined with input from the administrator and should be passed on through that vessel so staff knows they report to the administrator and s/he has blessed the message. A proper chain of command up and down the line.

Knowing that there is a defined logic to staffing is essential. It should go hand in hand with larger private practice groups. In some smaller groups, perhaps less so. But nonetheless, whatever group you happen to join, be sure that you do not have a situation where there are favorite staff members; sure we all like people who we get along with and having a great technician might be well and good, but staff who circumvent the office organizational structure do a disservice to your management team and, ultimately, your business by undermining and minimizing management.

As you can see below, as we regurgitate our org chart, there is a quasi-logical flow of decisions and a chain of command which should theoretically allow MDs to disseminate a plan, and that course of action passes down the variety of command lines to the appropriate individuals for implementation. Another telling component of the group's structure, physician disposition, and overall joy imbued by the MDs in the practice is how long the administrator has been employed. He's usually top dog on staff. At this point in the book, I'll tell you 2 things (caveats, if you will): first, I am a recovering administrator. So this comes from the heart and the trenches. Second, I feel like I know you well enough and can safely convey to you with some experience and insight that being an administrator, even in the best of groups, can be very, very trying. Remember, we're the folks who need to juggle the regulations and demands of a medical group *concurrently* with the business demands of the group.

## FUN/EDUCATIONAL ANECDOTE NUMBER 8

An associate recently was having a discussion with his managing partner. The discussion apparently became a bit heated when the managing partner uttered the following: " . . . it's not that big of a job . . . " as he referenced the administrator's job. To my way of thinking, this is not only insulting to the administrator but displays a clear lack of understanding of what it takes for the administrator to run the business.

To offer you a comical feel for the administrator's job description, please note the fabricated, but not too far off the mark, help wanted ad below that was offered by an associate. We operate in a bizarre business model with the need to keep multiple bosses (partners, shareholders, whatever you might call them) happy while striving to maintain staff, negotiate reimbursements to decent levels, and generally keep the ship afloat. Visions of the Dutch boy and the dike are probably not too far removed from the reality of day-to-day practice administration. The thing to keep in mind is that this business model is one that is highly complex. It is a business, in many cases a multimillion dollar business, and is fraught with the perils that running a small business carries. But to add a dimension of complexity and fun (he offered tongue-in-cheek), it is also one of the most regulated businesses in the country. And there are a perpetual 45 million uninsured in the country. (A number that I've not seen change much since 1990; so, could one make the argument that since there were roughly 248 million people in the US in 1990, and there are 300 million now, on a percentage basis this isn't so bad? I mean, there is a decrease from 18.07% of the population uninsured to 15% uninsured. [I'm kidding. That's academic. Now you can be part of the solution.])

In any event, as long as the government is involved and desires to somehow offer every American health care coverage, a laudable but challenging goal, the practice dynamic will change due to the ripple effect set off by Washington, and the industry will continue to be a hotbed of rules, regulations, and intervention.

So, though there are many, many good administrators out there, they are hard to find and the good ones would give their eye teeth to run a good practice, because they seem to be a masochistic lot seeking absolutely no thanks and nothing but problems and issues on a day-to-day basis. As someone smarter than me once said, "If you want a friend, get a dog." Good advice for the administrator, an employee truly in the sandwich generation: sandwiched between staff and physicians.

## ADMINISTRATOR'S JOB DESCRIPTION (LONG VERSION/ABRIDGED VERSION)

SEEKING THE PERFECT MEDICAL PRACTICE ADMINISTRATOR.
We have a unique opportunity for a practice administrator. The practice administrator must be resourceful, energetic, and creative enough for the challenges of medical practice management. The practice administrator should have training and/or credentials as:

- Insurance, tax, human resource and anti-trust attorney
- Certified public accountant with expertise in corporate, partnership, and personal tax as well as pension management
- Social worker
- Travel agent
- Psychologist
- Trained negotiator experienced with third-party payers and employee management
- Financial planner/investment counselor
- Health and safety inspector with expertise in OSHA law
- Clinical knowledge of a physician
- Architect
- Computer technician
- Local area network administrator
- Recruiter
- Procurement and supply manager
- Human resources/personnel manager
- Chief financial officer
- Maintenance and building manager
- Telephone technician
- Collector/bookkeeper
- Banker
- Lobbyist
- The administrator will have direct experience or training in the above duties. In addition to the above, we are looking for some specific other characteristics that the ideal candidate will have. The candidate:
  - Will be compassionate and supportive, but firm and decisive

- Will demonstrate superb leadership skills, which will motivate individuals to move mountains, without being authoritative
- Will have skills and experience as an excellent mediator and consensus builder including bringing agreement between 2 or more diametrically opposed points of view
- Will be able to prove that the age-old adage was incorrect and that it is truly possible to make all the people happy all the time
- Will have wisdom enough to make decisions like Solomon, to be humble enough to give all decision-making credit to others for positive results, and be willing to accept all culpability for decisions that have gone awry
- Have public speaking skills of an orator that are likely to inspire the masses, but friendly and down-to-earth enough to casually discuss last night's basketball game
- Will be able to communicate to people as an "average Joe" while maintaining a vocabulary and the word usage of a college English professor
- Will have personality traits that allow the candidate to be laid back enough to take stress with ease, but remain compulsive and controlling enough to manage a thousand details with intensity
- Able to prepare a clear and concise agenda for meetings with 5-minute notice
- Will demonstrate the integrity and compassion of Mother Teresa, while maintaining the business tactics and strategy of a railroad baron
- Will be able to accurately predict the future without mentioning any gloom-and-doom comments
- Will be able to prioritize and multi-task an infinite number of issues and projects based on the changing perceptions and needs of 5 or more physicians at a time
- Will be an involved community leader that spends quality time with their family without sacrificing long work hours
- Will possess the intelligence and education of a scholar while accepting the pay of a student

Or, put more narrowly:

ADMINISTRATOR JOB DESCRIPTION
Looking for a candidate to be all things to all people all of the time, regardless of the time. Candidate should:
- Know all and be infallible and,
- Master "all things" including, but not limited to:
  1. IT, HR, legal, med/mal, construction, contracting/negotiating, etc, and things NOT included herewith, and
  2. all things.

The administrator functions on a broad-reaching continuum, handling, in some manner or form, everything from employee issues to med/mal issues. They negotiate payer contracts on your behalf and look out for the best interests of the practice, **your** business. And, if I may be so bold, the administrator seldom if ever gets the old pat on the back. They are the prototypical 50s-era, *Leave it to Beaver* mom who is around, unobtrusive, making sure the house functions for Ward and the boys. If all goes well, that's the way it should be. If the proverbial pile hits the fan, then it all falls to Joan. Basically, when she's doing her job, you never know because she operates with such skill and acumen. See what I mean?

Administrator longevity in a practice is a good thing, if the administrator is good, capable, and plugged in to his/her specialty. If s/he is a muttonhead, then not so much. A long-term administrator shows continuity of management, displays the investment in institutional knowledge, and shows leadership and buy-in by the physician-owners. Someone at that level who has been with the practice for some time has either been shown the love or has been beaten into submission and has no alternatives available. You need to divine which is accurate for each and every practice you're going to. By the bye, "showed the love" equals the administrator is loved, is treated like a professional, and the MDs love the job that the administrator performs.

Running a medical group is, at its best and most optimal, a hard, oftentimes thankless job, but it offers the certain masochist the prospect of operating in a multi-tasking setting, experiencing HR, IT, medico-legal, to name but a few, simultaneously. A good, solid administrator will also have a feel for what it is you, as an MD, do. If you're a family practice MD, the administrator will understand the dynamics of family practice medicine, what a history and physical looks like in your setting, and some components of what you treat. There's a defined dichotomy in being an administrator: you're there to help the business and to grow the practice, and yet from time to time you need to manage and discipline your bosses! It's one very bizarre scheme in a decidedly bizarre industry.

Now a brief word to the wise. Don't look at administrators as a cost. Good ones will, year over year, find efficiencies, savings, and potential revenue streams that should come close to covering their salaries. In addition to that, they run a multimillion dollar business. You can, though you shouldn't, shortchange yourself on who's minding the store. It would, again, be shortsighted and detrimental to the business.

## FUN/EDUCATIONAL ANECDOTE NUMBER 9

So, a friend of mine in the business calls me and tells me he's been offered a proposition. He is in a fair-sized group (more than 10 MDs) in a specialty that is exceedingly demanding based on multiple medical modalities (there's alliteration for you) and, given the type of specialty, fraught with rules, regulations, and oversight apropos of their procedures. So, deservedly, he makes a good wage. His managing partner proposes a nifty idea. He suggests cutting the administrator's salary by what amounts to 99.99%. Hmm. Odd, you say? You'd be right. The idea was that the administrator would start a side business, keep all of the net profits, and work for the practice for $1 which, it would seem, would enable him to keep benefits. Well, this administrator, we'll call him Stunned, calls me to chat and recount this neato, yet very disturbing story. Stunned tells me this and, after picking my lunch up from the floor, I console him at the sheer insanity of the plan. Not only that, the business that was suggested was one in which Stunned could easily go out and start on his own with no assistance from the practice. Now, to the managing partner's . . . er . . . .credit(?), he's looking to save money and he probably thought that his idea was a sound one, in that it would enable Stunned the opportunity to expand his income while the practice saved some money. But taken a bit more pragmatically, had the managing partner reviewed this with some inkling of thoughtful deliberation, he'd have seen that a.) he just, in absolute terms, devalued the job that Stunned was doing, b.) offered Stunned nothing, really, that he couldn't do himself, and c.) basically just ticked Stunned off to no end. And Stunned's a good guy. It's a case of the MD not fully realizing all that goes into running the business, *his* business, of which Stunned receives NO equity and no value aside from a salary (not commensurate with the heartburn and crap) and a good effort.

## JEFF, WHO'S LEFT AND WHY DO I CARE?

If you're joining a small practice, say 2 or 3 docs, you'll have a very flat organization chart. It'll most probably be the owner or 1-2 owners and then an office manager or administrator. Many times, smaller groups are still managed by staff members who've come up through the ranks and, with due respect to them, are more suited to managing the business than running the business. Think of it, if you will, in terms of the front desk employee who has been with the group for 25 years but who is not really a manager. S/he is more of a technician in a manager's body. In these situations, the manager has received no formal education, has no credentials to run the group aside from longevity, and may not manage people well. The MDs may have grown the group but not the management infrastructure, so the tech who's been with Dr Z forever becomes, by default, the administrator. I'd ask the group about the administrator's background and, as we've said before, longevity. An administrator outside of his scope and skills is a recipe for problems and something for the new physician to keep an eye on in his/her job search.

That's not to imply that folks who've worked their way to the top of the food chain are not solid. But a majority of those folks, I'd argue, have their base talents surpassed by the speed with which health care now moves. Many of these folks find the management equation difficult and challenging, with too much to do, too much going on, and only the skill set to stay singularly focused vs multi-tasking.

As an MD in this type of small group, you'll handle things that will throw you, 0 to 60, into the trenches. You're smart so you'll learn, and you'll learn by fire. It's bad, because you were put on this earth to see patients and cure the ills of the world, after a fashion. And every moment you spend trying to run the practice is 1 less hour you spend in patient care or with your family.

If you join a large group, you'll major in patient care and minor in business stuff. This is good and it is bad. It's good because you were put on this earth to see patients and cure the ills of the world, after a fashion. It's bad because you do not get the trial-by-fire mentality of a small group struggling to survive. You'll need to decide which model works best for you.

In larger groups, as we've noted in the org chart, you'll have staff handling a variety of components for you; you'll have a more robust organizational architecture. You'll most definitely have a CEO-type who looks out for the bigger picture. You'll probably have a COO-type who handles the operational components. In this day and age, you'll decidedly have some sort of chief information officer (CIO) or Director of IT. CIO is a fun job to do on the side in a small group, but in a larger group, it's a job that an administrator/CEO cannot handle. It simply gets too complex and there are not enough hours in the day to handle it appropriately.

Additionally, if you're in a large group, you may have a Research Director (if you're heavy into clinical research and/or trials) and you'll have some sort of director of clinical operations or a managing RN. This person, or this role, is crucial, in my opinion, to carrying out the MDs clinical aspirations and assuring that care protocols are delivered and the follow-up that exists is sound, therewith closing the clinical care loop and assuring you've delivered appropriate care that has been followed by qualified staff.

If you're in a large group, you'll have a fairly good-sized billing office. Folks might be segmented by payer type or job function, and will work on getting the charges out and the money in. The person running this group must be familiar with coding in your specialty and is normally, in larger operations, a certified procedural coder (CPC, as mentioned earlier) and understands all of the complexities inherent in your specialty (multiprocedural surgery reduction for surgeries performed on the same day, for instance). S/he manages the charges going out, and the money coming in. They manage the insurance company rejections and the appeals. And no matter the size of your group, you'll want them keeping a careful and deliberate eye on the dollars going out and in. I feel, and this is just perception (see the newspaper clippings in Appendix 1 of this book), that some of the commercial payers in the world (meaning nongovernmental, like Medicare and Medicaid) may relish the fact that they can game you at every turn and reject claims (as delineated in their contracts, "dirty" them, if you will), presuming that you will not be able to meet the timely filing requirements of your contract if you wish to appeal. Is this an unfair assertion to level at unnamed payers? Maybe, but I don't think so, based on history. This is anecdotal, but it happens. There's no smoking gun, but there are a few shell casings. After being in this business for so many years, I've seen and heard things you would not believe in terms of payment avoidance, denial of claims as "trial" when the FDA had green-lighted modalities and drugs, etc. Generally, and only generally, the insurance companies are not your friends. So, having someone on top of this process, a dedicated person who knows what they're doing, is essential. You'll see the results of some of these commercial payer shenanigans as we address payers later on.

## SUMMARY

The take away message is that there needs to exist some structure, some skeleton, of the group you're interviewing with. As I've said before, this offers you another sign that some thoughtfulness and contemplation was afforded the group to move it forward in a planned way, as opposed to by happenstance, offers a sense of job function (reduces duplication of effort, inefficiency), and lends itself to flow throughout the organization.

Of course, if you're joining a smaller group or solo practice, there may exist very little structure to the organization. Nonetheless, there will need to be a defined role for you to play, both as an employed MD and as a partner. What's your role?

## OUTSIDE'S AS IMPORTANT AS INSIDE

The group is only as good, or as bad, as the counsel received from those professionals the MDs trust. For instance, most private practice groups do not employ an internal accountant or are not really large enough to have a staffed chief financial officer (CFO) position. The business size and complexity simply may not warrant the higher level and higher price-tag individuals. Some larger groups have a multitude of "C-level" professionals on staff to manage, with the senior physicians, the day-to-day operations of the practice. There are, believe it or not, private practice groups of greater than 50 physicians, which necessitate a fairly robust upper-level management structure not unlike a medium-sized corporation. Time to put on your business hat: a 50-physician group, depending on specialty, *could* generate upwards of $40-$50 million in revenue per year. So, that's a pretty good-sized little business. This set-up is not dissimilar to a regular corporation, and as such, you should look at this as a business. And their organization chart (as referenced on page 51) may be complicated by another layer of management within the organization. So, a word to the wise. I'd consider a multi-doc group of significant size (maybe greater than 15 physicians) that does not have at least a CEO-type to be understaffed in upper-tier management. This may be shortsightedness by the MDs (turf protection?), may mean the MDs play too large of a day-to-day role in managing the group, or that the MDs constrain the purse strings too much. In any event, none of the aforementioned scenarios bodes well. There's simply too much work to be done in a 15-MD group to *not* have a very robust upper-level management structure.

## *Accountants*

Most groups don't need one of the Big Four accounting firms to handle their taxes. But you do need qualified counsel to let you know how to run the books in your entity, which is structured as one of the corporate designations described earlier (PC/LLC). Better still would be an accountant with experience with medical practices, so they could explain and you could understand the ins/outs of the accounting approach. Most medical practices operate on a cash basis vs an accrual basis. Essentially, just so you know and for your edification, cash basis and accrual basis are essentially timing distinctions on when transactions are accounted for on the business's books. Most medical practices (general) run on a cash basis, meaning that you don't account for your revenues and expenses until they hit your books. Most other businesses outside of private practice health care use the accrual method of accounting. Under the accrual method, transactions are counted when the sale is made, the item is delivered, or the service occurs, irrespective of when the money for the services is received.

If you're looking at a smaller group, or even a larger one that employs the services of outside firms for advice, inquire about those firms. Find out about the accountants, how long the practice has been with them, and how many medical clients that accountant has. It would not be bad to know if they have a national presence or a local presence. If the group's administrator is a CPA and does the group's taxes, I'd still ask that an outside firm take a look at the taxes. It never hurts to have another set of eyes review the books to make sure that everything's on the up and up.

## *I'll take one lawyer, Alex*

The prior paragraph was certainly an entrée into this topic. What I said for accountants, ditto times 4 for attorneys. They, like MDs, like most people in life, come in different stripes, shapes, and sizes. The one thing I'd counsel is: make sure the practice you're getting involved with has good legal counsel in a variety of arenas. As I've said, and will say throughout this book, health care is a very highly regulated and monitored industry. It is still a $2.2 trillion, that's right TRILLION with a T, dollar industry annually. Ponder that for a sec. And yet, as someone smarter than me has said, it's a cottage industry. That is, it is not as sophisticated as many other business segments, because its focus is on health care, not the *business of* health care. So there's room for error there, no? And that's what doctors are bred for, is it not? To treat patients and focus on medicine. That's why fine folks like me have jobs. To help run the business. Likewise with the lawyers. The health care climate is getting more and more complicated on a daily basis, with subsets of health care law popping up seemingly daily.

As you perform your job search, I'd inquire of the group if they have attorneys who are knowledgeable about general corporate contract law, Stark, anti-kickbacks, antitrust, human resources, and HIPAA. There are larger firms who've developed a coterie of services germane to these topics, but you, and your new group, may need to shop outside of these subsets of law to assure you have received seasoned counsel on same.

Health care law has morphed over the last 15-20 years, mainly due to a few bad apples. To be quite fair, some unsavory clinicians have mucked up the works for future generations by cutting bizarre and self-serving deals that lined their pockets. As with most things, the government acted, then overreacted, and not unlike a pit bull, once they got their teeth into the soft underbelly of health care, they didn't let go. As is often the case, the government gets involved, oftentimes overzealously, and the result is a web of complex legislative mandates designed to penalize the few that instead actually penalize the lot. A leader in this business of what's good for health care is the fine California Senator Fortney (Pete) Stark, D-California, 13th District. Since his early attempts at reining in health care waste and abuse, Mr Stark has become the poster child for the body of law known as the Stark Law, which basically prohibits a physician from referring patients to entities in which the physician has a financial relationship. Many of us in the business have come to affectionately refer to the law simply as Stark. The Stark statute actually became effective in 1995, but the initial final regulations were not deployed until nearly 6 years later in 2001. Subsequent regulations have also been adopted. You can surmise how complex this law is.

In any event, and so as not to get bogged down in all that Stark entails, it is safe to say a little cottage industry for health care lawyers evolved, we'll call this a specialty, revolving around how to deal with Stark and work within its parameters.

There also exist federal anti-kickback laws that prohibit the referral of patients in exchange for the payment of remuneration to the physician.

After Stark and anti-kickbacks, or really in concert with Stark and anti-kickbacks, there is the ever-present HIPAA (phonetically "hipa"), The Health Insurance Portability and Accountability Act. The Act's name fits nicely into the government's need to craft a cutesy acronym for every law that they foist upon you. This law is just another weight that will hang around your neck until you're done practicing medicine. It's theoretically a government-imposed noose divined out of abuses in the system, specifically the sale of patient-specific information by certain entities in the early 90s. Basically, the crux of HIPAA is founded in some very solid and foundationally strong premises: that peoples' health records should be kept private and confidential. I have no problem with that. And if the government had constructed a 1-sentence law saying, in effect, "Now be it understood that patients' medical records are to be kept confidential," I'm sure that would've passed House and Senate without a beat. Instead, HIPAA was, as most bills are, loaded down with any form and measure of "stuff," emboldening the federal government to increase its domain over health care.

HIPAA simply (*really* simply) means you can't talk about a patient's medical record with anyone except the patient or a designee, and can share medical information with other medical professionals relative to the patient's care. It's laudable in that regard, and would probably be admirable if it was limited in that scope. But, as with most things governmental, it wasn't. And so, in the beginning it was a bear to manage and understand, its advent leading to yet another subspecialty of law.

The new practice you join should have a HIPAA Privacy Policy in place and should review it at least semiannually to assure that it's up to date and functional in terms of its requirements on the practice and staff, and that it continues to be implemented and monitored as a dynamic tool.

In addition to the federal laws listed above, each state has its own laws and regulations for health care, such as Certificate of Need (CON) laws, privacy laws, and self-referral laws.

The group you join should also have counsel steeped in the ever-shifting field of human resources law. This assures that rules and regs are followed and that you have a resource to go to if you need questions answered with regard to your staff. Remember, not only are you a medical office but you are a business and you employ people. As such, you're open to both state and federal regulations vis-á-vis employees. Even large practices, with a designated HR Manager (or a seasoned HR person) should have counsel to go to with questions. For smaller practices, it's essential.

*Qui tam and tam qui*

I mentioned *qui tam* lawsuits a little while back. Basically, a *qui tam* suit is a whistle-blower suit, which means that someone in your group sees something amiss with how the government is being billed and goes to an attorney to rectify this. This move of selfless sacrifice does not necessarily derive from a pure heart. Instead, many such suits are brought by disgruntled employees looking to stick it to their bosses (or former bosses). Some *qui tam* suits have been very lucrative for the plaintiffs and their attorneys. If a business (say a medical practice) loses a *qui tam*, the reporting whistleblower stands to receive between 15%-30% of the settlement. As you can see, there's some motivation for staff to turn you in. And, really, rightfully so. The message here is twofold:

make sure that you are billing governmental entities appropriately and, if you find a problem with same, or staff brings up an issue, be sure you (or your practice) addresses the issue post-haste.

## *No free lunch!*

Nothing is free. This harkens back a bit to Stark. Just so you know, you are not allowed to receive a free trip to Aruba in exchange for referrals. Anytime you're presented with something free, run, don't walk. It is illegal for you, generally, to receive gifts of value to influence your business. Any gifts should be *de minimus* in nature.

There are certain legitimate arrangements among referring MDs that can be addressed, but these creations require very careful analysis with your *qualified* health care attorney.

This is an area in which you don't want to skimp on qualified (read health care edu-macated) counsel. If deals are being struck, from the most complicated to the easi-est, having good counsel on board for a review is worth its weight in gold.

Let's look at another no-no. You can't own a piece of equipment and let MDs or clinicians who are not a part of your group (eg, same tax ID or other recognized rela-tionship) use it for free. It's considered by the government to be a possible induce-ment to refer. That is, if you have a Shmogamacolit, and Dr Z doesn't have one but Dr Z is an internal med doc who sends you patients (or could), and you let him use your Shmogamacolit while you're out of the office on Tuesdays, he uses it and bills for it. You think, fine, I'm not using it. But the government looks at it, as a Shmogamacolit costs $100,000 and Dr Z uses it for free. There's an implied thought that his referral patterns might be impacted by his ability to use that machine for free. Get it?

Hum this little ditty, like Dorothy in the *Wizard of Oz*, and you won't go wrong: "There's nothing for free, there's nothing for free, there's nothing for free."

So, as you can see, good counsel, covering a variety of topics, is a good thing to have, especially in health care.

## *Fair market value (FMV)*

And then there's your counsel on other items relative to law. For instance, if you're going to rent space from an MD, you must do so at a FMV rate to show that the deal benefits neither party untowardly. You cannot pay a premium to rent space, as it may appear to be, and in all probability is, an inducement to refer. Let's look at it this way. Ophthalmologist 1, call him MD 1, wishes to rent space from an optometrist, OD 1. MD 1 desires space 1 day per week, all day, because it seems in his estimation to be more cost-effective to rent space 1 day per week than it does to open, equip, and staff a new location full time only to use it 1 day per week. He knows that the business just isn't there yet and he'd like to test the waters before making a firm commitment to renting his own space. So OD 1 says he'll rent MD 1 some space, as OD 1 has some extra capacity (read: more time on his hands than patients). MD 1 and OD 1 must come to an agreement as to what the space is worth. That is, what the FMV is. Here's where you need to pay attention. Let us say that OD 1 pays $5,000 a month in rent for his space. If MD 1 needs one day per week, then the calculating may look (in its simplest form) something like this:

$5,000 rent

Divide by 30 days (1 month, even though one could make the argument there are only 20-22 working days a month; this is negligible)

$5,000/30= $166.67 per day

Renting one day a month, provided MD 1 has exclusive run of the place, should cost him about $166.67 per day or roughly $666.67 per month (4 days/month x $166.67). Now, one could also make a legitimate, FMV argument that a pro rata share of other fixed costs, such as electricity, renting equipment, etc, could be thrown into the mix. And this could be defendable.

Let's say now that the costs and assumptions above are static. But OD 1 wants $2,500 per month from MD 1 for MD 1 to get access to the space. Innocently, MD 1 *might* go ahead and do this, again deducing that at this price it is still less expensive to get into this arrangement than it is for him to get into a full 3- or 5-year lease somewhere else. Here's the rub. If the government were to look at this arrangement, they would wonder why MD 1 would pay half of OD 1's rent monthly for only 4 days worth of time in that office. They would most probably look at this as MD 1 paying OD 1 a premium so that OD 1 will refer Lasik patients, or general ophthalmology exams, or what have you, which is illegal. They would deem that MD 1 was helping OD 1 offset his costs and he would show his gratitude by sending patients to MD 1. MD 1 is deemed, ultimately, to be paying for patients. See?

The moral to the story: if a deal is set up with a referring practice and you lease a space in another practice, make sure you pay a FMV. You cannot simply go into his satellite office and pay his entire monthly rent. If you've not already been told, there are no free lunches. That applies to medicine. Really. There's nothing free in health care and anyone offering you anything more than a Bic pen is either not up to snuff on the law or is looking for something in return.

How about this scenario: Company Y sells Medicine 1. Company Y makes its living off of Medicine 1, as that's its only product line (the FDA dragging their feet and all). Now, Medicine 1, to be efficacious in the treatment of bicep bunions, must be deployed using Glue Gun 2000. A rep for company Y tells you that you can "borrow" Glue Gun 2000 for as long as you like. Interestingly, Glue Gun 2000 allows you to use more Medicine 1 in the process. See how that works? This looks good to you because you need Medicine 1, Glue Gun 2000 costs $50,000, and it is the key to deploying Medicine 1. If you can get it for free and dispense Medicine 1, why not, right? Wrong.

Of the general counsel for the group, I'd at least find out how long the attorney has worked with and for the group. Find out how long he has practiced health care law. If he has not, does anyone in his firm?

*Advisors, charlatans, and toe jam experts*

From time to time, there'll be a job, a challenge, a project that may be out of the purview of the administrator. After all, s/he is expected to be expert on all things but, truth be told, cannot be. In a busy medical practice, especially a very large medical practice, there simply is no time for the administrator to develop a defined knowledge on everything that is out there in the ether. So, from time to time, it'll be necessary to hire a consultant. There are good consultants out there and there are bad consultants out there. Just like there are good MDs out there and bad MDs out there. I mean, someone went to Bora Bora's Medical Institute for Healing and now practices medicine in the States, right?

I tend to shy away from consultants who do not have a history either in a health care practice (eg, have not run a practice. Look, if you've never done colorectal surgery, I don't expect you to teach a class on it!) or, at the very least, in their chosen specialty. Do not, emphasize NOT, hire a consultant just because he's friends with the Senior Partner. It would, or at least could, be a very bad move. You're not shucking corn here. You are in a highly regulated industry that requires experience (on the consultant's side) and very, very careful deliberation. There are many hoops to jump through in health care.

For example, let's say you're looking to build an ambulatory surgery center (ASC). There are rules and regs, some federal, some state-specific, about time to build, cost to build, location to build, etc. Just because the Senior Partner's buddy built a series of outhouses for the governor does not mean that he knows a darn thing about building ASCs. To expound on that, even if he does his research and learns all he needs in order to build an ASC, the costs could be far more than if you'd hired a firm and consultant or management advisor who'd done this in the past and has a history, either nationally or regionally, but preferably on a state level.

I'd vet consultants to an extent proportional to the complexity and involvement of the task at hand. For instance, if I'm looking at someone to help me with my accounts receivable, I might look at a couple of folks, ask their experience, ask for references, and ask to see/hear about results and improvements attained. If I were looking to build an ASC, or purchase and install an electronic medical record (EMR) system, I'd develop a series of questions and a request for proposal (RFP) and ask for multiple bidders on this project. The questions should be detailed, maybe bordering on painful for the bidders, as you will make a significant investment in the project (think 6-7 figures) and will need to know every skeleton about the vendors who are bidding and their ability to deliver on the promise. The last thing you want is to be $500,000 into an EMR installation and find out the bid did not include a fluxcapasitori-radiosternide-cablioblastinatious or two at a cost of $500K each. Then you'll learn the value of a good RFP process and having a good vendor.

Personally, I like consultants or advisors who've been in groups, either run them or run a segment of their specialty (eg, a CPC for coding issues and, even better, for your specialty-related coding issues), as this displays to me a very acute understanding about how the job they do impacts, and is impacted by, the office environment. Consultants with no practical experience have nil to zero experience of their ideas in the trenches, where the rubber hits the road, and they can just as easily be in, put their plan in action, and then move on to the next project without looking back, regardless of the results and the carnage left behind. Now, I know that consultants need good results to get future business, but some manage to survive, even thrive, in a sea of mediocrity buoyed by truly lackluster performance without a ding to their armor. They simply ride into the sunset, looking for the next dragon to slay.

If working with a consultant, I'd ask for measurable, quantifiable results. They should be happy to put in writing what they think they can attain. If done, this will assure that they keep a conservative expectation of what they can deliver.

*Outsourced stuff*

Some practices will outsource some or all of their human resources function or another component like their profit-sharing plan. Due diligence here can go a long way. HR is fairly generic. That is, what applies to one business generally applies to another, save for some state differences. So an HR firm can probably handle all you need, soup to nuts. But it's worth knowing their track record. This, however, should not impact how you look at the practice in terms of buying or employment.

## GOING ONE STEP DEEPER

Ok, let's recount. You've looked at the geography, the MDs in the area, and you've interviewed at a few places. You understand some basics regarding the organization chart and who manages what and whom. You know that the skills of outside counsel matter and that it's important to have qualified experts leading you and your team forward.

Now we're going to go one step deeper, down near steerage, near the engine room, where the staff fires up the engines and keeps the ship moving forward. We're going to look at coding.

Though this is, due to sheer volume and scope, going to be an abbreviated look at coding and billing, it should help give to you a basic understanding. Remember, the nature of this book is not an encyclopedic knowledge of practice and practice management, from A-Z. I want to give you a basic understanding of what you'll step into in your next life and put you one step higher up on the curve than your predecessors who learned by blood, sweat, and toil.

In general, in private practice, you get paid for billing CPT® codes. CPT® (Current Procedural Terminology), was developed, and is owned and trademarked, by the AMA. It is used and licensed by payers. The system has probably been a financial boon to the AMA in terms of revenue since its deployment some 40 years ago. In any event, CPT® codes tell insurance companies what you've done. Each code has a description. One code you may see a good bit of is the 99213, a "level 3" recheck code.

> *"**99213 Office or other outpatient visit** for the evaluation and management of an established patient, which requires at least two of these three key components:*
> *   *an expanded problem focused history;*
> *   *an expanded problem focused examination;*
> *   *medical decision making of low complexity.*
> *Counseling and coordination of care with other providers or agencies are provided consistent with the nature of the problem(s) and the patient's and/or family's needs. Usually, the presenting problems(s) are of low to moderate severity. Physicians typically spend 15 minutes face-to-face with the patient and/or family."*[3]

You substantiate a 99213 recheck by your documentation, which adds your reason for the level of service and ties in an ICD-9 (International Classification of Diseases - Volume 9), offering you the diagnostic reason as to why you performed a level 3 office visit. For instance, Patient X might come into the office to see you for continued care of his psoriasis. You might bill 99213 with an ICD of 123.45, "psoriasis undefined left quadrant of face." (By the way, this ICD-9 description, as far as I know, is fake.) You would then submit these codes to Patient X's insurance company and, in theory, you would get paid accurately and in a timely fashion for the procedure, based on an agreed-upon, prenegotiated fee schedule.

There are thousands of CPT® codes out there. This is certainly not the venue for getting into the rigors of how, when, and why CPT® codes are added and changed. A wonderful resource is the AMA's own Web site, at http://www.ama-assn.org/ama/pub/category/3882.html, which delineates in great detail how the process works. Suffice it to say, this is the coding component many of you will work under at least in the near term. AMA's annual CPT® 2010 *Current Procedure Terminology* is a great guide chocked full of codes and detailed descriptions.

## CPT® RANGES (GENERAL)

CPT® codes fall under these general ranges as listed in the *AMA's Guide to CPT Coding*: Evaluation and Management (E&M), Anesthesia, Surgery, Radiology, Pathology and Lab, and Medicine.

Later we'll go into the CPT® experience and what it might mean to you in terms of revenue and productivity, in a manner similar to how we defined what revenues you might contribute to the practice earlier in the book.

For now, though, let's look at the process. You bill your code. You do so electronically. Medicare is required to adjudicate claims filed electronically within 14 days of receipt. Commercial payers, depending on contracts and state laws, can generally take from 15-45 days to pay clean claims. Claims are oftentimes denied or rejected for a myriad of reasons. It's important to assure that staff in the billing area of the business remain on top of the denials. They should review all claims that come back through the office, check to be sure that reimbursements are what the practice had negotiated in its contract, minus co-pays, deductibles, or patient responsibility. If the correct amount was not paid for the service, staff should research and appeal the claim with all haste.

I like to see billing folks cross-trained but specializing. That is, I like to see a "poster," someone who logs the payments received into patient's accounts, focused on that component but knowledgeable about the accounts receivable person working on commercial (eg Aetna, BC/BS) denials. The reason for that should be obvious, but what I hope to achieve by such a set-up is to have the poster with specialized knowledge and therewith efficiency so that s/he can see problems that arise, payments that were less than they were supposed to be, and look for patterns and problems. If an issue arises, s/he can then move the issue to the billing manager (in a larger group) or an administrator to discuss the pattern and go to the payer for some response, resolution, what have you. The cross-training piece is important, because I believe it offers the poster some insight into other jobs in the billing/collections cycle, which enables them to fill in, even if temporarily, should someone be out of the office for an extended period of time. Cross-training assures that you don't miss a beat when a staff member is out. It's also a fairly elusive goal.

There are some groups who farm out the billing component altogether. I'm not a big fan of this. It can work for some groups and is cost-effective, but does not work for others. Now there's an adroit statement for you! But it goes to show that one size does *not* fit all for medical practices, and you need to find that balance. Whether or not to farm out billing is an individual decision to be divined by the MDs and administrator as to the value (cost savings) vs expense of losing absolute control over the process.

With the billing staff, there should be protocols in place to handle the claims. Many insurance companies (a leader of which is Medicare) offer electronic remittance advice and direct deposit of their funds. I'm a huge fan of this, because it gets your money in the bank a few days earlier, minimizes paper, and minimizes human intervention. How? You submit your claims. Medicare adjudicates them and issues back to you, electronically, advice on each claim. Some practice management software even auto-posts to patients' accounts, which means staff simply needs to review the remittance advice to assure that the money hit the right account in the right amount.

## ACCOUNTS RECEIVABLE

Accounts receivable, or AR, are the dollars outstanding due to the practice. These are usually broken down into "buckets," such as 0-30 bucket, 31-60 bucket, 61-90 bucket, and 91 and higher. The more AR in the 0-60 day buckets, the better the practice is doing in terms of collecting money due them. Too much money over 90 days could mean a lack of attention to the AR (eg, no process in place to handle AR), which translates into extra cost (eg, refiling, employee time spent chasing down money due the practice), and reduced revenues. According to the Commercial Collection Agency Section of the Commercial Law League of America[4], you are likely to receive 93.4% of money due you for bills 30 days out, 85.2% for bills 60 days out, and 73.1% for receipts out 90 days. Put differently, if you filed a $100 (net) charge, and you let that charge sit for 90 days, you might expect to receive $73.10. After 90 days, as you might surmise, the percent of collectibles does *not* increase. Not so good, eh? Though your collectibility in a medical practice may vary, I'd suggest that at best it doesn't improve by much over time. So, while how much you collect is important, how quickly you collect what is due you is nearly as important.

Net AR is defined pretty basically as the amount of money outstanding minus contractual adjustments and write-offs. It is the true dollar amount that you might reasonably expect to collect. That is, it is the amount of money the practice expects to collect after all adjustments have been taken. A contractual adjustment might look like this. You contract with Insurance Company 1 (IC 1) to provide new patient exams for $100. But your charge for that service is normally $150. When you bill Patient X for his visit, a patient with IC 1 as his insurance company, you will collect a $20 co-pay from Patient X at the time of service, and then you would bill IC 1 for the visit, and IC 1 would reimburse you $80. You would have received your contracted reimbursement (a $20 co-pay from Patient X added to the $80 reimbursement from IC 1 = $100) for that procedure, but you've charged $150 so you need to write off or adjust the remaining $50 of your usual and customary charge. If IC 1 has not paid you yet, you have $80 in net AR.

Let's look at another AR example. In the chart below, Drs X, Y, and Z have, for the period in question, an AR of $350,000. This, though, may not represent their net AR. Why? Because of that $350,000 outstanding, you don't know how much must still be adjusted due to write-offs and other contractual allowances. That's because most groups do not bill the expected fee schedule amount. They bill their charges, as we discussed earlier in the book. So, while you might hope to collect all $350,000, you may just collect a percentage of the $350,000 that is outstanding.

| Physician | CHARGES | RECEIPTS | ADJUST-MENTS/ WRITE-OFFS | OUTSTAND-ING AR | |
|---|---|---|---|---|---|
| Dr X | $1,000,000.00 | $800,000.00 | $100,000.00 | $100,000.00 | |
| Dr Y | $1,250,000.00 | $900,000.00 | $200,000.00 | $150,000.00 | |
| Dr Z | $1,400,000.00 | $1,000,000.00 | $300,000.00 | $100,000.00 | |
| | | | | $350,000.00 | Practice's outstanding AR |

*Collection ratio*

This leads us into our collection ratio. Our billed and collectible money might be broken down into a couple of categories. The gross collection rate, which entails the collections divided by the gross charges, and the net collection rate, which entails the collections divided by our gross charges *minus* our contractual adjustments. The net charges, synonymous to net AR, are what we should reasonably expect to collect.

A practice's gross collection ratio is seldom if ever employed, as it basically has little meaning. Net collections have value and should be on the order of 95%-100%.

Let us assume that Drs X, Y, and Z have figured that, over time, they have a 92% collection ratio. If we apply that figure to their outstanding AR listed above, we find that they may reasonably expect to collect $322,000 of that $350,000 outstanding, or 92% of the outstanding AR. This is useful, in that it enables the group to examine money on the books that should flow through the doors, meaning better budgeting and cash management.

Let us now look at Dr Fred Mendit Group, PC. As you can see, they had a decent year of charging out $7.56 million. They collected $6.94 million and adjusted off $561,000. They have an ending AR balance of $450,000. During the course of the measured 12-month period, they divined that they collected 99.65% of money due them. The tricky part about this exercise is that it is a picture in time, as with most data points. For instance, in January of 200X, the group had an AR of $400,000. They charged out another $600,000. They wrote off $45,000 and had an ending AR of

| Physician | CHARGES | RECEIPTS | ADJUST-MENTS/WRITE-OFFS | OUTSTAND-ING AR | |
|---|---|---|---|---|---|
| Dr X | $1,000,000.00 | $800,000.00 | $100,000.00 | $100,000.00 | |
| Dr Y | $1,250,000.00 | $900,000.00 | $200,000.00 | $150,000.00 | |
| Dr Z | $1,400,000.00 | $1,000,000.00 | $300,000.00 | $100,000.00 | |
| | | | | $350,000.00 | Practice's outstanding AR |
| | | | Net collection %: | 92% | |
| | | | Collectible money: | $322,000.00 | |

$405,000. They collected 99.10% of what they expected to collect for the month. But here's where it gets a little odd: their charges minus adjustments and write-offs (net charges) are $555,000. But those are for the month. The *payments* that came in may have actually been from charges posted the month or months before. So the group collected 99.10% of its collectibles for the month, but not of what was collectible *and generated* in that month. See?

As you can see, as highlighted at the bottom of Exhibit 6, the collections percentage for the preceding 12-month period is 99.16%, an *astounding* collection percent. To add, though not as accurate a measure, our gross collection percent of 91.80% is pretty stinking good, too.

A really good collection rate might go hand in hand with our next AR-related topic, the days in AR.

## DAYS IN AR

Days in AR is a measurement of how long it takes the practice to collect the money that is owed to the business or how long, on average and measured in days, your AR stays on the books. As you might intuitively surmise, an AR collection rate of 99.16% might indicate a pretty good days-outstanding in addition to good days buckets.

There are several ways to look at days in AR and to calculate same. The key to this exercise is employing consistency when reviewing these numbers, so that if there exists huge swings in values, you can begin to trace back to the root cause. If you change your methodology in your calculation, you run the risk of getting data that's decidedly skewed and returns very little value.

In the attached spreadsheet, we'll take Dr Mendit's Group and the same data that we looked at for his collections ratio. Now we'll examine his days in AR by taking the

**EXHIBIT 6.**

Fred Mendit Group, P.C.
January 1, 200X - December 31, 200X

Accounts Receivable, 1/1/200X - 12/31/200X

| | Starting AR | Charges | Payments | Adj/WriteOff | Ending AR | Collection % | Charges less adj/woffs |
|---|---|---|---|---|---|---|---|
| 1/31/200X | 400,000.00 | 600,000.00 | 550,000.00 | 45,000.00 | 405,000.00 | 99.10% | $555,000.00 ←collectible money |
| 2/28/200X | 405,000.00 | 625,000.00 | 525,000.00 | 35,000.00 | 470,000.00 | 88.98% | $590,000.00 |
| 3/31/200X | 470,000.00 | 675,000.00 | 575,000.00 | 55,000.00 | 515,000.00 | 92.74% | $620,000.00 |
| 4/30/200X | 515,000.00 | 600,000.00 | 550,000.00 | 55,000.00 | 510,000.00 | 100.92% | $545,000.00 |
| 5/31/200X | 510,000.00 | 600,000.00 | 600,000.00 | 48,000.00 | 462,000.00 | 108.70% | $552,000.00 |
| 6/30/200X | 462,000.00 | 650,000.00 | 600,000.00 | 45,000.00 | 467,000.00 | 99.17% | $605,000.00 |
| 7/31/200X | 467,000.00 | 550,000.00 | 625,000.00 | 42,500.00 | 349,500.00 | 123.15% | $507,500.00 |
| 8/31/200X | 349,500.00 | 675,000.00 | 625,000.00 | 48,000.00 | 351,500.00 | 99.68% | $627,000.00 |
| 9/30/200X | 351,500.00 | 650,000.00 | 595,000.00 | 45,000.00 | 361,500.00 | 98.35% | $605,000.00 |
| 10/31/200X | 361,500.00 | 680,000.00 | 575,000.00 | 40,000.00 | 426,500.00 | 89.84% | $640,000.00 |
| 11/30/200X | 426,500.00 | 660,000.00 | 550,000.00 | 50,000.00 | 486,500.00 | 90.16% | $610,000.00 |
| 12/31/200X | 486,500.00 | 600,000.00 | 575,000.00 | 52,500.00 | 459,000.00 | 105.02% | $547,500.00 |
| | | 7,565,000.00 | 6,945,000.00 | 561,000.00 | | | |

GROSS collection %: 91.80% — what you've collected relative to what you've charged
NET collection %: 99.16% — what you've collected relative to what is collectible

last 6 months of charges and dividing that number by 182.5 (1/2 of a year). The outstanding AR in the last period is then divided by the dividend of your prior calculation, yielding your days outstanding. As we can readily see, based on this calculation, the days in AR are an amazing 21.96. It is taking Dr Mendit's group about 22 days to collect money due them. As a point of reference, anything under 35 days is pretty darn good. Conversely, a days in AR of 90 means that it takes, ***on average***, nearly 3 months for the practice to collect monies due. That does not take into account the fact that you enter into the cycle of losing cents on the dollar for every day the collectibles languish in the buckets. Money you'll never see again.

If you want to dazzle your prospective employer, ask the managing partner, or better still, the administrator, how much of their AR is over 60 days old, what their net collection ratio is, and what their days in AR are.

Even if they are unwilling to offer you exact dollar numbers, the percentages, and the fact that they know them, is salient. That is telling without yielding too much information.

As an added bonus in Exhibit 7, we've put, in the far lower left hand side, a fictional sample of what percentage of the billed claims are in which bucket. Again, as one might imagine, a fair percent of the claims outstanding are in the 0-30 day bucket. Another good chunk is in the 31-60 day bucket. The other buckets are nice and low, meaning we're effectively managing the old stuff and keeping the new from growing old and becoming uncollectible. Like any business, you want to know how quickly the money is coming in.

As someone with a somewhat jaundiced look at payers, the insurance companies don't mind at all that you have a high AR and poor collection ratio. In fact, if they knew about it, I suggest to you they might be overjoyed. Why? Because it means that you have no idea how much money you're missing out on and have holes in your billing processes while they, in turn, do not need to pay out in a timely manner, meaning they keep their money and make money off of that money.

Working on these things and having a good back office is very important to cash flow. Ask your prospective employer if s/he has staff in place to effectively manage the incoming cash to the practice. Many practices short change this area in terms of staffing, as they think it's a waste of money. They look at it as a cost rather than an investment. But I can tell you stories of dedicated staff collecting multiple 6-figure sums simply by being dedicated to making sure that money due the practice was collected, either previsit (by verifying insurance due for certain procedures) or post-visit by diligently tracking money owed the business.

## CASH CONTROLS

Ask your prospective employer about their cash management procedures. Do they use a lockbox, where patient payments are mailed directly to the bank? Do they have good checks and balances in place to manage actual cash transactions at the front desk, like collection of co-pays or petty cash? Many are the war stories of practices that neither manage nor monitor the cash that changes hands, even at the front desk. This can

**EXHIBIT 7.**

Fred Mendit Group, P.C.

Accounts Receivable, 1/1/200X - 12/31/200X

January 1, 200X - December 31, 200X

| | Starting AR | Charges | Payments | Adj/WriteOff | Ending AR | Collection % | Charges less adj/woffs |
|---|---|---|---|---|---|---|---|
| 1/31/200X | 400,000.00 | 600,000.00 | 550,000.00 | 45,000.00 | 405,000.00 | 99.10% | $555,000.00 |
| 2/28/200X | 405,000.00 | 625,000.00 | 525,000.00 | 35,000.00 | 470,000.00 | 88.98% | $590,000.00 |
| 3/31/200X | 470,000.00 | 675,000.00 | 575,000.00 | 55,000.00 | 515,000.00 | 92.74% | $620,000.00 |
| 4/30/200X | 515,000.00 | 600,000.00 | 550,000.00 | 55,000.00 | 510,000.00 | 100.92% | $545,000.00 |
| 5/31/200X | 510,000.00 | 600,000.00 | 600,000.00 | 48,000.00 | 462,000.00 | 108.70% | $552,000.00 |
| 6/30/200X | 462,000.00 | 650,000.00 | 600,000.00 | 45,000.00 | 467,000.00 | 99.17% | $605,000.00 |
| 7/31/200X | 467,000.00 | 550,000.00 | 625,000.00 | 42,500.00 | 349,500.00 | 123.15% | $507,500.00 |
| 8/31/200X | 349,500.00 | 675,000.00 | 625,000.00 | 48,000.00 | 351,500.00 | 99.68% | $627,000.00 |
| 9/30/200X | 351,500.00 | 650,000.00 | 595,000.00 | 45,000.00 | 361,500.00 | 98.35% | $605,000.00 |
| 10/31/200X | 361,500.00 | 680,000.00 | 575,000.00 | 40,000.00 | 426,500.00 | 89.84% | $640,000.00 |
| 11/30/200X | 426,500.00 | 660,000.00 | 550,000.00 | 50,000.00 | 486,500.00 | 90.16% | $610,000.00 |
| 12/31/200X | 486,500.00 | 600,000.00 | 575,000.00 | 52,500.00 | 459,000.00 | 105.02% | $547,500.00 |
| | | 7,565,000.00 | 6,945,000.00 | 561,000.00 | | | |

← collectible money

GROSS collection %: 91.80%   what you've collected of what you've charged

NET collection %: 99.16%   what you've collected that is collectible

% in older AR buckets should, in theory, be low
as the days in AR are, on the aggregate, farily low.

| 0 - 30 | 50% |
|---|---|
| 31 - 60 | 35% |
| 61 - 90 | 10% |
| > 91 | 5% |

459,000.00

21.96   days in AR

happen in the smallest or the largest groups if no controls are in place. I've often been amazed at how innovative crooks can be. Had they dedicated equal time to performing their jobs, they probably would have been very successful at them. But I digress.

Let us look at it this way, very simply. Say you join a practice with 5 locations. Those 5 locations see 40 patients per day. That means the business has 200 patient encounters a day (5 x 40). Let's just say, for simplicity's sake, those 200 visits are simple office visits with $20 co-pays. So you are looking at $4,000 per day coming into the practice in co-pays, many times in credit cards but oftentimes in cash. Now, your practice may be open as many as 253 days per year, taking out weekends and 8 holidays. Given these assumptions, you could be dealing with nearly $1,012,000 in co-pays! That changes things a bit, doesn't it? And if just 10% of that comes in cash, that's roughly $101,000 changing hands annually. (See Exhibit 8.) Without good cash controls in place vis-á-vis checks and balances, that's a good opportunity for some unsavory check-in or check-out person to siphon off some

**EXHIBIT 8.**

| Fred Mendit, PC Examination of Co-Pays | |
|---|---:|
| Locations: | 5 |
| Patients/location per day: | 40 |
| Patient visits per day: (practice-wide) | 200 |
| Average co-pay per patient: | $20.00 |
| | |
| Revenue/day in co-pays: | $4,000.00 |
| Working days per year: | 253 |
| | |
| Co-pay revenue per year: | $1,012,000.00 |
| | |
| Assume 10% in cash: | $101,200.00 |
| Assume 90% in credit cards: | $910,800.00 |

of your hard-earned money. Does this happen? Yes. But oftentimes you don't hear about it, because physicians don't like to look foolish, and so the offender is normally fired and the matter dies away quietly. But I think you see where I'm going. You're not dealing, on a day-to-day basis, in nickels and dimes. In many practices, millions of dollars change hands annually.

## MARKETING

Most practices don't have a marketing person dedicated full time to marketing the group. That job normally falls on the office manager or administrator with help from a lead MD. In other words, most practices actually do have a marketing person, whether it's the administrator (jack of all trades, master of none), or, in a larger group, a designated person.

Marketing is not a 4-letter word in health care. At least not in my opinion. I believe that, tastefully done, it has a place, but it must be done so in very stark confines with parameters that are not always well defined. Before embarking on a major marketing campaign, I'd make sure that what I'm doing and the language I'm figuring to deploy is run by *qualified* counsel, to assure that I've not walked into a mine field with regard to promises and/or commitments that cannot be met and that open the practice up to legal and/or financial peril.

For example, you run an ad in Paper XYZ. You say, "We offer the best care available in treatment of chronic halitosis." Aside from the fact that this is probably factually incorrect, it is also making a claim that you cannot quantify and thereby cannot live up to. This is a pitfall that is akin to what we'd mentioned in your mission statement earlier in the book. It opens you up to considerable risk. As a takeaway, you should always, in marketing, take pains to avoid quality statements because, since medicine is the balance of art and science, it is equally difficult to measure quality.

To gauge the success of a marketing campaign, though, I might do something like this. You have a halitosis treatment that's been on the market. You want to advertise this elective procedure, where elective means, clinically, that the procedure is not necessarily needed but that the patient might elect to have the procedure done. Elective also usually means that the patient will pay out of pocket and the patient will not utilize insurance.

The procedure employs a laser that costs $100,000. We'll assume that all other costs for the life of the laser, to keep our example simple, are $25,000. You expect to generate $250 for each case. That means, to cover all costs over the life of the laser, to break even and generate a profit, we must perform 500 procedures. You already know that you cannot pay anyone for referrals or offer kickbacks as we've addressed this previously and at this point you are a legal scholar on all things health care.

Now you need to market the procedure. The problem is, you've never run an ad campaign before.

Word of mouth is always your best and least expensive marketing tool. That is irrespective of whether you're performing fancy-shmancy laser procedures or just seeing patients. This is because, if you deliver good care, give your patients more than the time of day, and listen, truly listen to them, they will be delighted. A delighted patient will tell friends of their great experiences. As an aside, there is an anecdote that if you delight 1 person, they may tell 4 people. As the adage goes, if you anger 1 person, they may tell 10. The adage "the customer is always right" is not necessarily dead-on, but it sure hits the target near the bull's-eye.

Back to our example. You decide to market the new procedure. You can make that fact known. The procedure is new to the area and you're the only Board Certified Whatchamacallit doing Chronic Halitosis Laserflageroptomy. Let's get moving.

First, I would identify potential candidates within the practice. I'd data-mine our computer system to see which patients I have who might fit the criteria and mail a direct ad piece to them. Better yet, I'd flag those people as they came into the office and let them know of the procedure as I move it forward. I'd put posters up in the waiting room and in the exam rooms. And I'd train the staff on the new procedure, its benefits, and let them help in the internal marketing. We get the front desk team in each

**EXHIBIT 9.**

| | |
|---|---|
| Laser cost: | $ 100,000.00 |
| All other expenses: | $ 25,000.00 (over the life of the laser; includes marketing budget) |
| Total cost: | $ 125,000.00 |

| | |
|---|---|
| Break even: | 500 (how many procedures will need to be done before the laser is paid for itself) |
| Payment per procedure: | $ 250.00 |

| | |
|---|---|
| Procedure slots in a year: | 1000 |

| # of patients from Ad cycle 1 | | # of patients from Ad cycle 2 | | Cost per pt. cycle 1 | Cost per pt. cycle 2 | Cost per pt. cycle 1 | Cost per pt. cycle 2 |
|---|---|---|---|---|---|---|---|
| 10 | radio | 15 | radio | $ 50.00 | $ 33.33 | $ 500.00 | $ 500.00 |
| 1 | t.v. | 0 | t.v. | $ 1,000.00 | $ - | $ 1,000.00 | |
| 6 | print | 25 | print | $ 16.67 | $ 44.00 | $ 100.00 | $ 1,100.00 |
| 0 | word | 10 | Word | $ - | $ - | $ - | $ - |
| **Total:** 17 | | 50 | | | | $ 1,600.00 | $ 1,600.00 |

Cost to convert 1 pt to a "sale:"  $ 94.12 | $ 32.00

office set up with some sort of method to identify how folks have heard about the new procedure. A simple spreadsheet.

Let's now look at the cost of marketing. We'll do an ad buy for radio, TV, and newspaper. Say in the first cycle ad campaign our TV ad buy is $1000 for the month. (We're assuming all ad buys are for 1 month only.) Our radio ad is $500 and our newspaper ad is $100. We plan to spend $1,600 on our marketing in ad cycle 1.

We've run our ads. How do we know what is working? Well, you can begin to aggregate the data from the folks calling in. Exhibit 9 offers an idea.

What we find is that it has cost us $1,000 *per patient* to get a person in via a TV ad, $16.67 per patient to convert a patient via newspaper ad, and $50 to convert a patient from a radio ad. At this point, we've had no one come in via word of mouth. And overall, it cost us $94.12, on average, to get a patient in the door to have the procedure done. Now, at $94.12 per patient, on average, it would take you a good long time to pay off that laser.

What we now have, though, is some baseline data. We know that to get a patient on board via TV ads is neither economically feasible nor cost-effective. The cost to advertise in that way is *nearly double of what we receive to perform the procedure!* There's an old adage. If it costs you $10 to make a chair and you sell it for $9, you can't make up the deficit on volume of sales.

So we're now shifting away from TV ads. We'll examine very carefully if we obtain business through word of mouth. We know that we have happy customers and we want to know how that's going, so we'll keep an eye on how the word of mouth moves forward. In month 2, we've done away with TV and reapportioned our $1,600 budget to areas we know are working. We're going to give radio another chance and throw $500 toward that ad. We'll bump newspaper print to $1,100. Say in month 2 we get 25 people via newspaper ads, 15 via radio, and now 10 from word of mouth. This is how the ad money breaks down:

Your paper has gone to $44 and your radio to $33, but your 10 patients via word of mouth have, arguably, cost you nothing. I know there's a cost. I know that your ad buys heretofore probably got some of these folks thinking. But in broad terms, if Suzie Q had the procedure done and loved it, then she might've told Janie Q. And, Janie Q may *never* have heard of the procedure, until she'd spoken to Suzie Q about it.

So we now know that in month 2 our overall costs are approximately $32/patient to get a patient in the door and converted to a sale. We lowered the per-cost sale by keeping our marketing budget static and utilizing better advertising buys. And we know our word of mouth is growing by leaps and bounds.

What we've divined from this exercise is how to evaluate how our marketing dollars are spent and quantify the return(s) we've realized. This will better enable the business to market effectively in the future via avenues it knows are tried and true.

Marketing comes in different shapes and stripes. You can market via the method stated above, which requires little MD intervention aside from approving the plan and the clinical content, if any. Or you can market MD to MD. When you're speaking with your prospective new employers, I'd be interested in how much MD-to-MD outreach takes place. Do the MDs contact their referrers to touch base, to check on the perception of care given and the perception of patient time? This is something that, in part, can be farmed out to qualified management staff but isn't normally done. Here's the thing: MDs from other groups don't want to speak with another group's administrator. They want to speak with MDs. And to farm out entirely an important touch component like marketing to a staffer is generally not the best idea.

Another marketing avenue, as we alluded to, is patient satisfaction. Do not do a disservice to this component of the business. After all, the patient is why you're here. And delighting them should be your goal. But stating that you look to satisfy the patient and actually doing it may mean 2 different things. You may envision satisfaction as you restoring a limb. The patient should thank you profusely. But the patient may view satisfaction as a nice wait in the waiting room, cordial staff, reasonable accommodations in the office, and oh yeah, by the way, thanks for saving my limb. In other words, you performing your job does not necessarily translate into the patient having the time of their life in your practice and walking out the door with a feeling of satisfaction. So please don't delude yourself into thinking that patients are happy to wait 5 hours in a cramped, dank waiting room so that you can dazzle them. Their satisfaction has a great deal to do with their particular clinical outcome. But let us not be overly hubristic in thinking that we are the only clinicians out there offering limb reattachments, ok? I hope you get the bigger picture here.

## PAYERS AND SUCH

Ok, lots to impart here and limited space in which to do it. We'll get into some of the nuances of how to negotiate contracts with payers but I won't delve deeply into that science. Most of you will never experience that joy on a micro-level, but it can't hurt to be educated. We'll cover a few basics.

### Commercial/public payers

On this side of the fence, when we speak about commercial payers we are, in general terms, talking about the likes of UnitedHealthcare, Aetna, CIGNA, and the various Blue Cross/Blue Shield plans. These are some of the larger commercial players, among many, in the country. These include the for-profit and not-for-profit Blues plans, even though they generate huge sums of profits and return few of those dollars back to health care providers; go figure. The public payers are comprised of government-funded health plans, such as Medicare and Medicaid (Medicaid plans are federally and state-funded).

The commercial payers are corporations who, by and large, are in this business to make money. That's their job. They are put on this earth to, like Google or Coke, make money and return value to shareholders. Right off the bat, this is an interesting dichotomy apropos of health care, no? Look at it this way: government-sponsored plans are the public plans and the for-profits are the private plans.

### A few words about payers and profits

It never ceases to amaze how payers will try to drive down payments to physicians while increasing their own bottom line. Now, I understand the basics of the model. After a million econ courses, both undergrad and grad, I feel I kind of get the logic. But to drive profits at the expense of patients is downright criminal. (Not literally.)

The definition of profit from *Merriam-Webster* is: "A valuable return." "The excess of returns over expenditure in a transaction or series of transactions *esp* the excess of the selling price of goods over their cost."[5] As noted above, some of the largest commercial payers in the country include UnitedHealthcare, Aetna, and CIGNA.

United's 2008 revenues were a paltry $81 *billion*, returning a profit on the order of nearly $3 *billion*.[6] Aetna didn't fare as well. They had revenues of nearly $31 *billion* with reported profits approximating $1.3 *billion*.[7]

CIGNA earned a profit of about $292 *million* on revenues of nearly $19 *billion*.[8]

According to Atlantic Information Services, the CEOs of Aetna and CIGNA earned $24 million and $12 million, respectively, in total compensation for 2008.[9]

The bottom line is you'll need to glean an understanding of your customers. One group of which is the insurance company. And they'll run you through the ringer with one coverage decision after another, slips and changes to contracts that they'll mail to you (under obligation) which you'll miss in a pile of paper as you sort through your daily charts, notes to be signed, etc. The resulting effect of that memo, let's say, is on your imaging business. The commercial pay company is letting you know that they're cutting your reimbursements 10% or requiring preauthorization or what have you. In any event, "surprise" if you and your staff are not sophisticated enough to evaluate, change, adjust, and adapt on the fly.

That's why there exist software products to examine rejections (there are some out there that actually examine trends) and the need to have solid staff geared toward collecting all that is due the practice, and not just writing off an amount when the insurance company suggests the group has been paid all that is due. Knowing your contracted amounts is crucial.

## MEDICARE

Medicare is the child of the Centers for Medicare and Medicaid Services, or CMS. It is run by the Department of Health and Human Services. Though there's been some consolidation in the industry, Medicare farms out the day-to-day operations of its plans to carriers on the Part B side and intermediaries on the Part A side of the business. The carriers and intermediaries are insurance companies that handle one or more states and may adjudicate, or process, both Parts A and B claims. Part C is considered the Medicare Advantage arena, generally products that Medicare subs to commercial payers to administer the program for beneficiaries who carry Parts A and B Medicare. Part D is the drug piece of Medicare.

Sometimes Medicare carriers are at liberty to make certain clinical decisions on their own, within the parameters of the program mandates as issued from above. These are called local coverage determinations (LCDs), indicating what can and cannot be done clinically in a state or region.

One last, little, teensy-weensy item with Medicare. Medicare only covers items it deems "reasonable and medically necessary." So if you're performing a procedure on a patient that's either uncovered or deemed "not medically necessary," it will not be paid. Enough on that.

In the late 1980s, a team from Harvard developed the Resource Based Relative Value Scale (RBRVS) which Medicare began to unveil in a stepped approach beginning in 1992. Basically, Medicare envisioned physician expenses growing out of control. There was once a time when practitioners were paid based on the charges *they submitted!* For instance, I submit a bill for $150 for an office visit, I got paid my "usual and customary" payment based on my charge. Eg, if my charge was $150, I got paid 80% of the $150 while the patient paid 20% of the portion; their burden for utilizing health care.

## THE WORLD OF HSIAO*

*This will be boring but informational. Read it and like it. Thank you.

Dr Hsiao has been on the health care scene for a long time. A Harvard professor of Economics in the Department of Health Policy and Management, Dr Hsaio and his crew worked to develop a new pricing methodology for the federal government. Put basically, the scheme meant assigning weights and values to the AMA's CPT® codes based on certain criteria. Under Medicare, these criteria are updated annually in rather complex (remember, this book is about *facile*) gymnastics that adjust the values either up or down. Generally, just so you know, they're adjusted down. We'll look at how the values of codes are impacted by those machinations but will not dissect the logic, theory, or reasoning behind the RBRVS system. We could get into that, but I've probably already bored you to tears and don't wish to push you near suicide with an overly dry dissertation.

In any event, Dr Hsaio and company assigned values based on the work it took to perform a procedure, the possible malpractice exposure brought on by performing the procedure, and the cost to the practice in performing the procedure. In addition to this, realizing that geographic disparities in the costs to provide care from one location of the country to the next existed, Dr Hsaio and his team applied allowances for these differences. That is, to practice medicine in New York City might be more costly than it is in, say, Bum Shmoe, Iowa, so Dr Hsaio and his team realigned the reimbursements via Geographic Practice Cost Indices (GPCI, or, its cutesy government acronym, phonetically "gypsies").

So Dr Hsaio, by taking the values of procedures and adjusting them by geography, reasonably sought to pay physicians based on the work effort, med/mal exposure, and cost to the practice for performing each procedure in a given area.

Each value, work, practice expense, and malpractice expense is multiplied by the GPCI. Those products are then summed and multiplied by a standard, nationally applied conversion factor (CF) to give you the final dollar value of your procedure code. Pretty exciting, huh?

This is a lot to digest purely by reading about the calculations. If you're like me, you like seeing numbers on paper. I'm a visual kind of guy. So let's put this process into play and take a look at what this boils down to. Let's look at how you'll get paid by Medicare in the private practice setting. Medicare may play a significant role in your practice in terms of your patient mix and, subsequently, what the practice generates in revenues. Having said that, it wouldn't hurt you to have a general understanding of how Medicare pays you.

We'll look at your basic, run of the mill level 3 (mid-range complexity and decision making) recheck office visit, CPT® code 99213, (as defined previously).

The verbiage for this code was described on page 75. To determine what Medicare will pay for it in 2009, say, in the greater Atlanta area, we would employ the following calculation:

$$[(RVUw \times GPCIw) + (RVUpe \times GPCIpe) + (RVUmp \times GPCImp)] \times CF = fee^{[10]}$$

To see how area of the country (using the Gypsy) impacts the reimbursement, we'll look at the same office procedure comparatively between the greater Atlanta area and Richmond, Virginia.

As you can see by Exhibit 9B, the RVUw, RVUpe, and RVUmp remain the same, ostensibly because the work required in the procedure, the practice expense that is necessary in each practice, and the med/mal risk are static from location to location, state to state. However, the costs to perform the procedure, as indicated in the different Gypsy values, varies. In other words, and as you might intuitively surmise, it costs more to practice medicine in Atlanta than it does in Richmond, Virginia. This theory should hold true on most procedures.

This is a very simple look at how you'd be reimbursed by Medicare. There's much, much more to get into, and if our paths ever meet, it might be worthwhile to get caught up on this.

All of this said, does your practice need to calculate these reimbursement rates annually? Of course not. Medicare takes care of that for you. But it is worthwhile for you to know *how* to calculate these rates, so that you have an understanding of the components that comprise your reimbursement and you'll know, for instance, how to figure out the impact on your practice when Medicare says they are cutting the conversion factor for the upcoming year or that the work values are being amended via a budget neutrality adjuster.

Also, many commercial payers use some iteration of the Medicare fee schedule in negotiating reimbursements with physician groups.

## LASTLY, AS A DRY ASIDE

One thing that has heretofore impacted the reimbursements from Medicare is the ballyhooed Sustainable Growth Rate (SGR), which, according to Medicare " . . . is intended to control the growth in aggregate Medicare expenditures for physicians' services."[11] SGR's goal is not to withhold payments for physicians' services. In its

**EXHIBIT 9B.**

2009

Formula:

$$[(RVUw \times GPCIw) + (RVUpe \times GPCIpe) + (RVUm \times GPCIm)] \times CF = \text{Medicare Allowable}$$

| | | |
|---|---|---|
| Atlanta, Georgia | $[(.92 \times 1.009)+(.75 \times 1.014)+(.03 \times .836)] \times 36.0666 =$ | \$ 61.81 |
| Richmond, Virginia | $[(.92 \times 1.00)+(.75 \times .942)+(.03 \times .657)] \times 36.0666 =$ | \$ 59.37 |

**Level 3 recheck (99213) - Atlanta**

| RVU (Relative Value Unit): | RVU | |
|---|---|---|
| RVUw | 0.92 | "work" |
| RVUpe | 0.75 | "practice expense" |
| RVUmp | 0.03 | "malpractice expense" |
| GPCIw | 1.009 | "work" |
| GPCIpe | 1.014 | "practice expense" |
| GPCImp | 0.836 | "malpractice expense" |
| Conversion Factor (CF) | 36.0666 | |

**Level 3 recheck (99213) - Richmond, VA**

| RVU (Relative Value Unit): | RVU | |
|---|---|---|
| RVUw | 0.92 | "work" |
| RVUpe | 0.75 | "practice expense" |
| RVUmp | 0.03 | "malpractice expense" |
| GPCIw | 1.000 | "work" |
| GPCIpe | 0.942 | "practice expense" |
| GPCImp | 0.657 | "malpractice expense" |
| Conversion Factor (CF) | 36.0666 | |

arcane language, it is designed to look at expense targets set via mathematical gymnastics; if those targets, those actual expenditures for the program are exceeded relative to *projected* expenditures, then the update is decreased. That could mean a cut for Medicare reimbursements for the next year. (The SGR update for 2009, for instance, examined cumulative program expenditures from April 1, 1999 through December 31, 2008.) If expenditures are *less* than projected, which, by the bye, *never* happens, the update is increased for the coming year. This means reimbursements will receive a positive adjustment and should, generally, increase for the upcoming year. The SGR takes into account, as one of its components, real (inflation adjusted) gross domestic product (GDP). It has been argued by people immensely smarter than me that incorporating GDP into this convoluted calculus does not account for the fact that the economic activity measured by real GDP does not take into account the actual cost of providing care to patients.

This SGR thing is really just a heads-up. There are moves afoot as I write this book to amend or do away with it in calculating the Medicare fee schedule. However, if you're a glutton for punishment, if you are overly masochistic, you can find a real insomniac's dream, er, some salient facts regarding SGR on the Web at http://www.cbo.gov/ftpdocs/75xx/doc7542/09-07-SGR-brief.pdf. The document is entitled CBO Economic and Budget Issue Brief, September 6, 2006, p.2.

*So, how would Medicare cuts impact my practice?*

Great question. And you'll notice I did not ask how do Medicare *increases* impact your practice. In your practicing lifetime, whatever iteration Medicare and its payment schemes (d)evolve into, there is a very limited, let's call it a scintilla of a chance, that you will experience an increase in Medicare reimbursements on the aggregate. And if you do, that increase will be nominal, at best.

Oftentimes, the specialty societies (ACC, AAO, etc) will evaluate very proactively what the proposed cuts by Medicare entail and how those might impact, say, ophthalmology, on the whole. Yet the impact may affect you quite differently, dependent upon your patient mix and procedures performed. For instance, if your specialty society looked at a proposed fee schedule cut of, say, 21%, as has recently been suggested for 2010, would that mean your reimbursements would drop 21%? Not necessarily. They might drop even more!

The pain you'll feel is predicated on how much work you perform on Medicare beneficiaries and what **type** of work you perform on those clients.

Here's how we'll look at Medicare cuts that are slated to take place and how they might impact 2 fictional practices. Our little analysis will be performed on 2 ophthalmology groups practicing in the same area of the country (so as not to be impacted by Gypsies).

Dr X is a general ophthalmologist who performs a fair amount of cataract proce-dures, CPT® 66984. After learning in November, when the Final Rule is proffered by the federal government, that cuts for 2010 were on their way, Dr X's awesome prac-tice administrator, Awesome, culled his 10 most frequently used CPT® codes on Medicare beneficiaries from the practice's database and then aligned them by fre-quency in descending order. As you can see, Dr X's top 10 codes range from a high of level 3 consults (99243) to a low of a level 1 new patient visits (99201). Awesome arrayed his individual CPT® codes billed for 2009 in descending order by the number of times the code has been utilized. Plugging in the frequency of CPT® codes and multiplying that number by the fee for 2009 yields the expected reimbursement for 2009 for 99243, namely $4,734.52. Taking the same frequency of visits (projected for 2010) and apply-ing the proposed 2010 fee, you see the reimbursement expected to be $4,486.25.

**EXHIBIT 10.** Dr X Ophthalmology

|  | CPT code | Units YTD'09 | 2009 fee | Proposed 2010 fee | 2009 reimburse. | 2010 reimburse. | gain/(loss) Difference |
|---|---|---|---|---|---|---|---|
| 1 | 99243 | 37 | $127.96 | $121.25 | $4,734.52 | $4,486.25 | $(248.27) |
| 2 | 66984 | 25 | $712.13 | $636.22 | $17,803.25 | $15,905.50 | $(1,897.75) |
| 3 | 99203 | 25 | $101.22 | $91.24 | $2,530.50 | $2,281.00 | $(249.50) |
| 4 | 99242 | 22 | $95.96 | $88.44 | $2,111.12 | $1,945.68 | $(165.44) |
| 5 | 99204 | 20 | $142.85 | $138.17 | $2,857.00 | $2,763.40 | $(93.60) |
| 6 | 99205 | 18 | $181.15 | $173.07 | $3,260.70 | $3,115.26 | $(145.44) |
| 7 | 99255 | 15 | $201.63 | $190.69 | $3,024.45 | $2,860.35 | $(164.10) |
| 8 | 99202 | 9 | $68.12 | $61.88 | $613.08 | $556.92 | $(56.16) |
| 9 | 99252 | 8 | $74.45 | $71.74 | $595.60 | $573.92 | $(21.68) |
| 10 | 99201 | 5 | $38.55 | $35.76 | $192.75 | $178.80 | $(13.95) |
|  |  |  |  |  |  | Difference: | ($3,055.89) |

Awesome noticed that, *all things being equal*, if Dr X performed the exact same work on Medicare patients in 2010 as he did in 2009, the business would lose $248.27, or 5.24% on CPT® 99243, a mid-level consultation. In reviewing his top 10 codes, Awesome found that the business, all things being equal (assuming Dr. X sees the same Medicare patient mix in 2010), will lose $3,055.89 doing the same volume of work on Medicare clients in 2010 as he performed in 2009! This is a drop of nearly 8.1%.

Looked at slightly differently, if Dr X worked as hard on Medicare patients in 2010 as he did in 2009 he would LOSE $3,000.

Lastly, note what the cut in reimbursement means to Dr X's revenue on his cataract business, CPT® 66984. He will lose nearly $1,900, about 62% of his overall loss, if he performs the **same number of cataracts** in 2010 as he did in 2009. (Put alternatively, Dr X must now do 2.98 more cataract surgeries on Medicare patients to remain static.) Let's also say that Dr X's annual revenue for the entire business, including all payers, is $50,000 for 2009. If the proposed cuts are enacted, Dr X would experience a 6.11% *cut* in his business revenue performing the same procedures.

Now we'll take a look at Dr Y down the street. Same kind of scenario. Dr Y runs a good general ophthalmology business with very limited surgery. His decent administrator, Pretty Good, performed the exercise on his Medicare patient database that Awesome did above. Look at the results in Exhibit 11.

**EXHIBIT 11.** Dr Y Ophthalmology

|  | CPT code | Units YTD' 09 | 2009 fee | Proposed 2010 fee | 2009 reimburse. | 2010 Reimburse. | Gain/(loss) Difference |
|---|---|---|---|---|---|---|---|
| 1 | 99203 | 50 | $101.22 | $91.24 | $5,061.00 | $4,562.00 | $(499.00) |
| 2 | 99243 | 38 | 127.96 | 121.25 | $4,862.48 | $4,607.50 | $(254.98) |
| 3 | 99204 | 25 | 142.85 | 138.17 | $3,571.25 | $3,454.25 | $(117.00) |
| 4 | 99205 | 18 | $181.15 | $173.07 | $3,260.70 | $3,115.26 | $(145.44) |
| 5 | 99202 | 15 | $68.12 | $61.88 | $1,021.80 | $928.20 | $(93.60) |
| 6 | 99242 | 12 | 95.96 | 88.44 | $1,151.52 | $1,061.28 | $(90.24) |
| 7 | 99201 | 10 | $38.55 | $35.76 | $385.50 | $357.60 | $(27.90) |
| 8 | 99255 | 8 | 201.63 | 190.69 | $1,613.04 | $1,525.52 | $(87.52) |
| 9 | 99252 | 5 | 74.45 | 71.74 | $372.25 | $358.70 | $(13.55) |
| 10 | 66984 | 3 | $712.13 | $636.22 | $2,136.39 | $1,908.66 | $(227.73) |
|  |  |  |  |  |  | Aggregated difference: | $(1,556.96) |

As you can see, Dr Y really runs a pretty general medical ophthalmology clinic. He spends most of his time seeing new patients, consults, and rechecks, with a smattering of cataract surgeries (CPT® 66984) just to keep his hands in things, so to speak.

Again, Pretty Good arrayed, as Awesome did, in descending order Dr Y's top 10 codes by the number of times they were performed during 2009. Given the same geographic area but a slightly different patient mix, you can see that Dr Y is impacted differently than Dr X, his projected overall Medicare reduction is 6.64% or approximately $1,556.96. All things being equal, Dr Y will experience about $1,500 *less* in Medicare cuts than will Dr X. Also, Dr Y's practice should generate, in 2009, about

$50,000 in revenue. If the proposed Medicare cuts held true, he would notice roughly a 3.11% drop in his revenue. Lastly, notice, too, that Drs X and Y each performed 184 units during the measured period on Medicare patents.

In summary, both practices will now need to examine their patient base and their costs. Dr X might, for instance, divine that he can no longer accept new Medicare patients at those rates, as it will eventually drive him to bankruptcy. Or, he might keep doing what he's doing but let go of 2 staff members, team members he really needs as his paperwork continues to increase and the regulations continue to variously require more staff just to keep up.

*What are you, and your new group, going to do?*

The above examples, of course, are dependent upon variables that may be out of your control. For instance, the types of procedures you perform on the Medicare client base is dependent upon what patients present with. This is where medicine deviates from business; in the business world, a money-losing product line could be scrapped. In health care, dropping that money-losing line might entail no longer performing surgeries! That's one of the many odd dichotomies in this business model.

The take away message is that *your* Medicare reduction may or may not be the amount touted by some professional associations. The only way to gauge proposed cuts for any given year is for your Awesome and Pretty Good administrators to analyze your practice's Medicare procedures for the current year and apply the proposed fees to those numbers.

To stave off proposed cuts to the Medicare program, certainly physicians and their management teams should get involved with the process. This annual ritual usually begins early summer and runs until the government's final rule is published in November.

Physicians should get their management team (administrator) involved to contact national legislators (try to go through their local offices) and discuss with them your thoughts on the cuts and what those mean to you, your community, and your patients, especially given the fact that the cuts are expected to continue into the near future. Businesses should also assure that your administrator is running as efficient a practice as s/he can, scrutinizing how you spend your revenue.

It is often asked whether or not Medicare is at the breaking point. Are physicians leaving the program in droves? Actually, based on a recent Congressional Budget Office report, "More than 90 percent of physicians and non-physician professionals . . . participate in Part B."[12] (You'll recall that Part B reimburses physician offices.) The article continues stating, rather ominously, that "the situation may change if payment rates are significantly reduced."[13]

## COMMERCIAL PAYERS

And yet. And yet the cost to run the business continues to increase. The demands on the business (regulatory and other) continue to increase. What type of business model is this where, essentially, you provide the product (or service) and **don't get paid until days/months later!!?**

Try this as an analogy to the insanity of the business model you are now entering. Go to your grocery store this Saturday morning, run your groceries through the scanner, then tell the happy cashier that you'll be back in 15-30 days to pay for the groceries, at a discounted percent of the store's charges, of course, and you may not pay for some items, say the Nutter Butters and Trix cereal, because they may turn out to be unnecessary purchases for the household. See how that plan works for you. Not only that, consider what an associate of mine, Bill Hughes, sagely offered not too long ago. I think it hits the nail on the head relative to how patients view health care:

> "People will pay $350.00 for a stereo, but they wouldn't dare pay $200.00 for a physical . . . $125 a day to get into Disney per person, but won't pay a co-pay or a $50.00 lab test . . . $45,000 for a car that won't last over 6-7 years but wouldn't dare pay $2500 for out-of-pocket surgery."

Yet that is rather similar to what you'll do here and experience in health care. You will see a patient (provide a service), they will pay a fraction of the service provided that day (a nominal co-pay), you will submit the claim and wait to see if it is paid, denied, or more data is needed. In the meantime, if your billing folks are not savvy, the claim may be denied for services that were provided that were deemed unnecessary or the like. So, the patient/customer received the service at a cost to you of no less than a couple hundred dollars and you have, to that time period, received a $15-$50 co-pay, depending on the patient's insurance plan.

Commercial payers reimburse you physicians just a little differently than Medicare. There's normally much less ambiguity in commercial payer fees and fee schedules. I guess by ambiguity I mean you don't mess around with looking at RVU data to calculate your fee. Normally, a commercial payer will suggest paying you a percent of Medicare. For instance, a fee schedule might suggest that Private Payer X, we'll call them Moneybags, will pay you 120% of Medicare's fee schedule.

Paying as a percent of Medicare is all well and good given you understand how Medicare reimburses for services in your area. But since you've purchased and read this book, you now possess a basic understanding. Good for you.

What I like to do is look at the payers individually (eg, Aetna, BC/BS, UnitedHealthcare) based on the services we've provided for those patients during a calendar year, and see how they've reimbursed on the aggregate relative to Medicare. I would also bundle all

**EXHIBIT 12.**

| | NB1 $$$ | NB1 # of Procedure | NB1 Revenue | NB2 $$$ | NB2 # of Procedure | NB2 Revenue | Medicare 200X $$$ | # of Procs | 200X Medicare (MC) Revenue | NB 1 measured as a % of MC | NB 2 measured as a % of MC |
|---|---|---|---|---|---|---|---|---|---|---|---|
| 99202 OFFICE/OP E&M-NEW | $ 70.00 | 4 | $ 280.00 | $ 80.00 | 22 | $ 1,760.00 | $ 65.12 | 2 | $ 130.24 | $ 140.00 | $ 160.00 |
| 99203 OFFICE/OP E&M-NEW | $ 75.00 | 6 | $ 450.00 | $ 85.00 | 42 | $ 3,570.00 | $ 96.28 | 4 | $ 385.12 | $ 300.00 | $ 340.00 |
| 99204 OFFICE/OP E&M-NEW | $ 150.00 | 8 | $ 1,200.00 | $ 155.00 | 30 | $ 4,650.00 | $ 145.57 | 6 | $ 873.42 | $ 900.00 | $ 930.00 |
| 99205 OFFICE/OP E&M-NEW | $ 195.00 | 10 | $ 1,950.00 | $ 205.00 | 20 | $ 4,100.00 | $ 182.34 | 4 | $ 729.36 | $ 780.00 | $ 820.00 |
| 99212 OFFICE/OP E&M-EST | $ 40.00 | 12 | $ 480.00 | $ 45.00 | 100 | $ 4,500.00 | $ 38.72 | 2 | $ 77.44 | $ 80.00 | $ 90.00 |
| 99213 OFFICE/OP E&M-EST | $ 70.00 | 8 | $ 560.00 | $ 75.00 | 200 | $ 15,000.00 | $ 62.21 | 4 | $ 248.84 | $ 280.00 | $ 300.00 |
| 99214 OFFICE/OP E&M-EST | $ 98.00 | 7 | $ 686.00 | $ 105.00 | 180 | $ 18,900.00 | $ 94.21 | 6 | $ 565.26 | $ 588.00 | $ 630.00 |
| 99215 OFFICE/OP E&M-EST | $ 130.00 | 3 | $ 390.00 | $ 135.00 | 150 | $ 20,250.00 | $ 127.18 | 8 | $ 1,017.44 | $ 1,040.00 | $ 1,080.00 |
| 99241 CONSULT-OFFICE/O | $ 133.00 | 2 | $ 266.00 | $ 140.00 | 125 | $ 17,500.00 | $ 125.00 | 2 | $ 250.00 | $ 266.00 | $ 280.00 |
| 99242 CONSULT-OFFICE/O | $ 138.00 | 4 | $ 552.00 | $ 145.00 | 150 | $ 21,750.00 | $ 135.00 | 4 | $ 540.00 | $ 552.00 | $ 580.00 |
| 99243 CONSULT-OFFICE/O | $ 150.00 | 8 | $ 1,200.00 | $ 155.00 | 175 | $ 27,125.00 | $ 145.00 | 6 | $ 870.00 | $ 900.00 | $ 930.00 |
| 99244 CONSULT-OFFICE/O | $ 165.00 | 95 | $ 15,675.00 | $ 175.00 | 160 | $ 28,000.00 | $ 155.00 | 4 | $ 620.00 | $ 660.00 | $ 700.00 |
| 99245 CONSULT-OFFICE/O | $ 190.00 | 4 | $ 760.00 | $ 200.00 | 140 | $ 28,000.00 | $ 175.00 | 3 | $ 525.00 | $ 570.00 | $ 600.00 |
| 99252 CONSULT-HOSPITAl | $ 210.00 | 2 | $ 420.00 | $ 215.00 | 20 | $ 4,300.00 | $ 200.00 | 4 | $ 800.00 | $ 840.00 | $ 860.00 |
| 99253 CONSULT-HOSPITAl | $ 235.00 | 25 | $ 5,875.00 | $ 240.00 | 40 | $ 9,600.00 | $ 225.00 | 6 | $ 1,350.00 | $ 1,410.00 | $ 1,440.00 |
| 99254 CONSULT-HOSPITAl | $ 265.00 | 20 | $ 5,300.00 | $ 270.00 | 35 | $ 9,450.00 | $ 250.00 | 8 | $ 2,000.00 | $ 2,120.00 | $ 2,160.00 |
| 99255 CONSULT-HOSPITAl | $ 300.00 | 0 | $ - | $ 320.00 | 20 | $ 6,400.00 | $ 275.00 | 4 | $ 1,100.00 | $ 1,200.00 | $ 1,280.00 |
| | | | $ 36,044.00 | | | $ 224,855.00 | | | $ 12,082.12 | $ 12,626.00 | $ 13,180.00 |
| | | | Expected revenue from NB 1 | | | Expected revenue from NB 2 | | | % of 2007 Medica | 105% | 109% |

NB = Name Brand Private Payers
$$$ = reimbursement
# = # of times the procedure performed
** all rates are fictional and used
only for this example **

commercial payers to see what I get reimbursed for all payers on the aggregate. In many parts of the country, your commercial payers will pay more than Medicare. Again, this is predicated on your area of the country and your specialty. An example is in Exhibit 12.

The language in the contracts is generally straightforward but can hide landmines. Oftentimes, the language is set in stone, depending on your negotiating leverage. Remember that the contracts do require careful reading and an understanding of how each topic will impact the practice. There's no room in this book to cover contracting in its entirety, but I would suggest that the administrator and a lead physician review the contracts and be privy to their expiration dates. Most contracts are evergreen, meaning that they'll keep going, normally in 1-year increments, if not addressed prior to expiration.

From time to time, if the practice is willing to take the time, there may be some wiggle room regarding certain components of the contract. In theory these are negotiations. If a payer needs your group in their network, they may be willing to give more, whether it's via language or in the fee schedule. Remember that earlier in the book we discussed that a benefit of being part of a larger group was more leverage in contracting with payers. Going into these negotiations, you should know what you want to get from the payer and where you're willing to settle.

A key piece in the contract, in my guesstimation, is how you will be reimbursed. I'll keep this pithy and keep you from falling asleep. If a commercial payer is quoting you a contract as a percent of Medicare, you need to make sure you or your administrator knows what reimbursements for Medicare were for the year in question. That way, you can analyze how those fees will impact you in a manner similar to our Medicare fee cut example above. One thing to watch out for. Innocuously enough, some contracts state something akin to "115% of the Medicare fee schedule," which on its face may not be bad. I mean, you might be overjoyed that your largest commercial payer is willing to give you 115% of Medicare. But keep this in mind. If Medicare's rates go down the next year, and this contract is not renegotiated, what you were collecting from that commercial payer just automatically adjusted downward, too, as evidenced in Exhibit 13.

**EXHIBIT 13.**

If your private pay contract is tied in to Medicare rates for a given year:

| | Fee Year 2009 | Fee Year 2010 | Increase/ (decrease) | # OF TIMES PERFORMED | % Change in fee: +/- | REVENUE GAIN/ (LOSS) |
|---|---|---|---|---|---|---|
| MEDICARE: | $ 200.00 | $ 185.00 | $ (15.00) | 30 | -7.50% | $ (450.00) |
| PRIVATE PAYER: | $ 230.00 | $ 212.75 | $ (17.25) | 20 | -7.50% | $ (345.00) |
| | | | | You just took a | | $ (795.00) LOSS!!! |

What the figures above show you is that if your fee schedule is tied to a base Medicare year, like 2009 in our example, and the Medicare fee schedule drops 7.50%, you can see that your commercial payer fee schedule automatically adjusts downward as well. And, you can see that if you perform the exact same procedures in 2009 as you did in 2010 (eg, 30 for Medicare and 20 for the commercial payer), you would lose $450 with Medicare and $345 for the commercial payer, meaning you'd eat a total loss of $795 without a drop in your procedures.

So, if your payer is looking to offer a percent of Medicare, make sure, minimally, that the fee year is static throughout the contract's life. And, if you can, find the most profitable Medicare fee schedule in the recent past to use as your pegged fee schedule.

Alternatively, you might be able to work your fees based on a code-by-code basis, focusing on those CPT® codes which you perform most frequently. This might yield better results than an across-the-board fee schedule based on a percent of Medicare.

A non-exhaustive list of things to ponder in negotiating with commercial payers is your negotiating position (eg, do they need you in their network) and your data. You are at a decided disadvantage if you are negotiating and you are not willing to walk away or the commercial payer could care less whether or not you're in their network. You're business is only as good as your data.

Now, on with the show. So, is 120% of Medicare a reasonable rate for your services? Well, this may be good or bad, depending on where in the country you live and your specialty. For instance, some payers in some states actually pay *less* than Medicare (Part B), though most do not.

Your control over a market, as with any product, may dictate how much you can negotiate out of a payer in terms of their need for your specialty. It's a bit of basic economics as we mentioned earlier, supply and demand.

First, you get paid by submitting a "super bill," a sheet (otherwise known as a 1500, the gold standard in claim forms) either electronically or on paper, as we mentioned previously. You place your CPT® codes on the claim and append your ICD-9 codes. You submit your claim and wait.

As we said, many payers pay claims and send remittance advice electronically. That process is good for both parties to the system; you receive your money quicker (provided your claims are "clean" [billed appropriately]) and the payers get to cut down on paperwork and administrative costs associated with processing claims. Much of the process is handled without human intervention.

One last neat thing: in this crazy business, it is ok to for Medicare to publish what it will pay physicians and other clinicians throughout the country. They do so annually and are pretty good about keeping clinicians up to snuff about all things program related. On the flip side, however, you may not call your buddy in the same specialty down the road and say, "Make BC/BS pay you $1000 for splenectomies." That is collusion and is illegal. You are colluding to artificially inflate the price of the service and force the market to pay a higher rate than what it might otherwise have paid. Also, don't call your buddy and say, "If none of us sign this contract, they'll need to raise their rates." Again, this is colluding to keep a payer out of the market, is viewed as anticompetitive, and is patently illegal. Establishing fee schedules should be done in the individual practice and in accordance with the cost structure and practice needs. This book does not attempt to advise physicians on setting fees but points out methods that exist in the market place.

And along those lines, you cannot tell your buddy and his or her group not to take a contract so you can stick together. If you're separate groups, this too is illegal. Let's say your practice was right next door to the fine folks at the Department of Health and Human Services, the entity that heads the CMS. Just so you know, normally it is *verboten* to share fee schedule allowables under the Sherman Antitrust Act; this is viewed as anticompetitive. The logic is akin to BP and Exxon colluding to fix prices on fuel, if you will, or Coke, Pepsi, and Dr Pepper getting together in some back room to jack up the cost of a can of soda. Also, just so you know, Medicare's allowed to do this. Makes no sense, right? Of course. More on that later.

Such is the dichotomy in rule-making at the federal government. They can tell you, and other insurance companies, what they'll pay. Yet you cannot discuss how to set fees with your competition.

Disclaimer part of the show. I am not a lawyer. But this stuff is pretty shady. To learn how bad, call your health care attorney.

*Now wait a minute, Jeff, I charged a bazillion for that!*

As a basic heads-up, you don't get paid your charges. You'll get paid some adjusted value of them. We touched on this a little earlier in the book but more detail is now relevant.

Let us say, for instance, you might charge BC/BS $100 for an office exam, but BC/BS might contract with you to pay $90 and Medicare might contract with you (well, not really. There is no negotiating with Medicare) to pay $75 for the same procedure. The difference, in these instances, is adjusted to show that the claim was settled in full. You do not get the difference back. So, if you're looking at a group who tries to show you how busy they are by telling you they bill $8 bazillion a year, temper your enthusiasm against the reality that billing $8 bazillion per year may really only net you (eg, money in the door) $200,000. The charges really have NO impact on what commercial and public payers are going to pay you *save* for if the charge values are kept static year over year and are used as some sort of productivity measurement. This is if you charge $100 for an office visit in 2009 and charge $100 for an office visit in 2010, so you could look at charges as a *component* of overall productivity. But I would dissuade this measure, as most practices amend their charges. Insurance companies pay you either what you negotiated for your reimbursement (commercial) or what they've dictated, er, legislatively mandated they would pay you (public payers). The key is the net collectible charges or money the practice would reasonably expect to collect.

However, in your interview process, what you could do is look really sharp by asking Dr X, or Awesome, his trusty administrator, how much net revenue the business generated and how that matches up relative to peers inside and outside the group. Let Dr X know that his net charges are more telling than gross charges.

Let me explain charges another way. Fred Mendit, MD, is a surgeon, so his charges are pretty high. In 1 week, he sees no patients in the office and he performs 10 Igamagnectomies (my medical terminology) at a *charge* of $1,000 each, so his charges are $10,000 for the week. Seems good. I mean, if he takes 4 weeks off per year and performs the same number of cases each week (he's in demand and is the best surgeon he knows) he's working 48 weeks each year and generating $480,000 in charges.

Now let's look at Ignatious Schmoe, MD. Ignatious is in Dr Mendit's multispecialty practice but has decided to be a general physician, a shelf stocker, if you will, concentrating, in his waning practice years, purely on medicine. Dr Schmoe sees 10 patients a day in the same time period as Dr Mendit performs his 10 Igamagenectomies. Dr Schmoe charges $200 for these high-level consults (remember, this is for round numbers; if Dr Schmoe did nothing but code level 4s, he'd probably receive a call from his helpful Medicare fraud investigator!). So, back to the overly simplistic math: 10 patients a day, 5 days a week, at $200/charged per visit for 48 weeks. As you can see, Dr Schmoe has charged out the *same* dollar amount as Dr Mendit for the year-long period measured. But Dr Mendit receives, from Medicare, $600 for each of his Igamagenectomies, whereas Dr Schmoe receives, from Medicare, $190 for each level 4 office visit. So, all things being equal, Dr Mendit has generated $288,000 in revenue (on charges of $480,000) while Dr Schmoe has generated $456,000 (on charges of $480,000). Obviously charges, in this case, mattered not a whit and did **not** translate into productivity. You can see this in Exhibit 14.

**EXHIBIT 14.**

*Bazillion Dollar Charges - Who Cares?*

| Fred Mendit - MD | Surgeries per day | per week | Weekly charges @ $1000/ea. | | Annual Charges | Revenue/ submitted charge |
|---|---|---|---|---|---|---|
| Igamagnectomies: | 2 | 10 | $ 10,000.00 | $ | 480,000.00 | $ 288,000.00 |

| Ignatious Schmoe - MD | Patients per day | days/week | Weekly charges @ $200/ea. | | Annual Charges | Revenue/ submitted charge |
|---|---|---|---|---|---|---|
| Level 3 new patient: | 10 | 5 | $ 10,000.00 | $ | 480,000.00 | $ 456,000.00 |

Also, so you know, you might want to chat with your employers about their work RVUs, as aforementioned. It can be telling to know how many RVUs each MD produces or how many they produce relative to the peers in their specialty. I like to break that down on an MD-by-MD level, then apply the mean and median to those numbers. Why? Because Dr Hsiao's (remember him?) work RVUs are what they are and are a fairly static measuring tool, during any given year, of what people are doing. And so, if you look at his work values (even if they are not completely accurate or representative of actual work effort), they are basically consistent and represent the amount of work done by each clinician.

Ask your group-to-be if they track work RVUs and, if so, how far outside are the outliers from the median.

Many groups run 2 fee schedules. One for Medicare and 1 for commercial payers. The reason? Medicare fees are what they are. Yet if you charged only Medicare rates, you would lose money on all of your commercial payers. Some practices do this so that they do not have overinflated adjustments. This keeps the dollar value of their adjustments low. As you can see, in the example below, 2 fee schedules are deployed: 1 for Medicare and 1 for Name Brand 1 insurance, representative of our commercial payers. We charge Medicare the allowable, knowing that we will not receive more than the allowable. Thus, we look at the product of our procedures billed (the 1s) multiplied by the Medicare allowable. We see that our contractual adjustments are $0. However, with Name Brand 1, we see that we have charged a premium (our actual charges) and received our contracted rate. Going through the same exercise and math gymnastics as we did with Medicare, you can see that we adjusted off, based on our contract with Name Brand 1, $127.85. (Exhibit 15)

If you had 1 fee schedule in place, as in Example 2 within Exhibit 15 above, your adjustments would be higher, because you would need to adjust your Medicare charges, knowing that you would not receive from Medicare what you usually charge. As you can see, our contractual adjustments increase because we are writing off all of the adjustments that Medicare would not pay us. Using 1 fee schedule, 1 charge schedule, our adjustments increased from $127.85 to $620.81.

There really is no right answer to this question, just a matter of preference in terms of the practice's comfort and tolerance for adjustments.

## PAYMENTS AND SUCH

I won't bore you with the details and I'm no expert in this realm but, as we've said, Medicare must adjudicate your clean electronically filed claim within 14 days of submission, while most commercial payers have within 15-45 days, depending upon your state and the terms of your contract.

Truth be told, in terms of consistency and standards, Medicare should prove to be one of your more stable payers in terms of timeliness, refiling, etc. Commercial payers,

**EXHIBIT 15.**

Running two fee schedules v. one fee schedule

**Example 1 - Two Fee Schedules**

| CPT Code | # of Procedures | Medicare Charge schedule | Medicare Payments | # of Procedures | Name Brand 1 Charge schedule | Name Brand 1 Payments | Charge LESS Allowable |
|---|---|---|---|---|---|---|---|
| New patient visits | | | | | | | |
| 99201 | 1 | $ 37.48 | 37.48 | 1 | $ 60.00 | $ 48.72 | $ 11.28 |
| 99202 | 1 | $ 65.12 | 65.12 | 1 | $ 90.00 | $ 84.66 | $ 5.34 |
| 99203 | 1 | $ 96.28 | 96.28 | 1 | $ 135.00 | $ 125.16 | $ 9.84 |
| 99204 | 1 | $ 145.57 | 145.57 | 1 | $ 200.00 | $ 189.24 | $ 10.76 |
| 99205 | 1 | $ 182.34 | 182.34 | 1 | $ 250.00 | $ 237.04 | $ 12.96 |
| Consults | | | | | | | |
| 99241 | 1 | $ 50.88 | 50.88 | 1 | $ 75.00 | $ 66.14 | $ 8.86 |
| 99242 | 1 | $ 93.33 | 93.33 | 1 | $ 135.00 | $ 121.33 | $ 13.67 |
| 99243 | 1 | $ 127.67 | 127.67 | 1 | $ 175.00 | $ 165.97 | $ 9.03 |
| 99244 | 1 | $ 186.78 | 186.78 | 1 | $ 265.00 | $ 242.81 | $ 22.19 |
| 99245 | 1 | $ 231.59 | 231.59 | 1 | $ 325.00 | $ 301.07 | $ 23.93 |
| | | $ 1,217.04 | 1,217.04 | | $ 1,710.00 | $ 1,582.15 | $ 127.85 |
| Charges less collections: | | | $ - | Charges less collections: | | | $ 127.85 |

**Example 2 - One Fee Schedule**

| CPT Code | # of Procedures | Medicare Charge schedule | Medicare Payments | # of Procedures | Name Brand 1 Charge schedule | Name Brand 1 Charge MINUS Allowable |
|---|---|---|---|---|---|---|
| New patient visits | | | | | | |
| 99201 | 1 | $ 60.00 | 37.48 | 1 | $ 60.00 | $ 48.72 | $ 11.28 |
| 99202 | 1 | $ 90.00 | 65.12 | 1 | $ 90.00 | $ 84.66 | $ 5.34 |
| 99203 | 1 | $ 135.00 | 96.28 | 1 | $ 135.00 | $ 125.16 | $ 9.84 |
| 99204 | 1 | $ 200.00 | 145.57 | 1 | $ 200.00 | $ 189.24 | $ 10.76 |
| 99205 | 1 | $ 250.00 | 182.34 | 1 | $ 250.00 | $ 237.04 | $ 12.96 |
| Consults | | | | | | |
| 99241 | 1 | $ 75.00 | 50.88 | 1 | $ 75.00 | $ 66.14 | $ 8.86 |
| 99242 | 1 | $ 135.00 | 93.33 | 1 | $ 135.00 | $ 121.33 | $ 13.67 |
| 99243 | 1 | $ 175.00 | 127.67 | 1 | $ 175.00 | $ 165.97 | $ 9.03 |
| 99244 | 1 | $ 265.00 | 186.78 | 1 | $ 265.00 | $ 242.81 | $ 22.19 |
| 99245 | 1 | $ 325.00 | 231.59 | 1 | $ 325.00 | $ 301.07 | $ 23.93 |
| | | $ 1,710.00 | 1,217.04 | | $ 1,710.00 | $ 1,582.15 | $ 127.85 |
| Charges less collections: | | | $ 492.96 | Charges less collections: | | | $ 127.85 |
| Total contractual adjustments: | | | **$ 620.81** | | | | |

for whatever reason, seem to deny things, dance around the claims, and/or simply "dirty" claims. The logic seems to be that recourse, if taken, is long and drawn out.

One last thing. I'm not writing this book to bash payers. But I want MDs to know that, historically, payers have not been their friends. Below is an example of what I speak. For a couple further examples, please see Appendix 1 in the back.

This is but one of many items that has arisen during the last couple of years. So why, you ask me, do insurance companies shaft MDs? Well, my humble opinion is that they can. Look at the market caps (eg, what they're worth in the stock market) for

## Introduction

Welcome to the Blue Cross and Blue Shield Settlement website.

This website is intended to provide information to Class Members about the Settlement with the Blue Cross and Blue Shield Association and certain Blue Cross and Blue Shield Plans and certain current and former subsidiaries and affiliates in the class action lawsuit known as Love, et al. v. Blue Cross and Blue Shield Association, et al.

The Blue Cross and Blue Shield Association, certain Blue Cross and Blue Shield Plans and certain current and former subsidiaries and affiliates, who are participating in the Proposed Settlement are known as the settling "Blue Parties." For a complete list of the settling Blue Parties, please refer to the Documents page or to the Notice, which was mailed to Class Members on July 27, 2007 and which is included on this website. For a copy of the Notice, please click here: Notice

As used on this website, capitalized terms have the meaning ascribed to them in the Settlement Agreement

In order to qualify for a settlement payment, you must complete a Claim Form, sign the form, and mail the completed and signed form by NO LATER THAN OCTOBER 19, 2007 to:

Blue Parties' Settlement Administrator
PO Box 4349
Portland, OR 97208-4349

As described more fully in the Question and Answer (Q & A) section of this website, Class Members were mailed a Notice explaining their rights under the Settlement as well as a Claim Form and Claim Form Instructions on how to fill out the Form. This website includes those mailed documents sent to Class Members. Accordingly, Class Members should check for updates to this website to ensure that they have received all relevant instructions.[14]

---

United (UNH), Aetna (AET), and BC/BS (WLP). They are $33 billion, $12 billion, and $24 billion, at the time of this writing, give or take a few million. It would seem that if they need to pay out $30-$40 million in some settlement, where the attorneys stand to gain about one-third of that, and the plaintiffs, in many cases the physicians, gain pennies on the dollar, then it may be worth the fight. Besides, $30 million is a drop in the bucket. Ultimately, the MDs win nothing as the process to research the claims involved in the settlement is oftentimes more costly than the proceeds the MD might gain from the suit.

Given the aforementioned allegations, one might assume, if one were an assuming man, that some commercial payers basically "played the float" with money rightfully due MDs. They can fight and lose these legitimate lawsuits, but when you look at the market caps of United or Aetna, they can stand to lose a couple cases. And who wins out? Certainly the attorneys. I know it's a lot of work for them and they invest a good bit of time in these class action suits, but they seem to receive what anyone would call reasonable remuneration for such suits.

## REVENUE FOR A DAY

Earlier we looked at what you might expect to generate for the practice in a moderately conservative manner. It was hoped that that data might empower you to get a baseline feel for what you might, minimally, generate in revenue for your future employers. Figuring your potential revenue-generation for a practice is really fairly complicated, especially when there are ancillary modalities involved. What we'll do in this example is:

Assume Medicare is at least 1/2 of your overall business. Assume the remainder is made up of a hodge-podge of commercial payers, leaving the self-pay and/or indigent folks out of the equation to allow us to be fairly conservative.

I'd build a spreadsheet (which I can do for you) to show the following. We will not look at associated office-based procedures, such as injections, echos (ultrasounds), nuclear studies, CTs, etc. Instead, being conservative, we'll focus on our 50/50 office-based practice.

Your office visits are, basically 99201-99205 for new patients. We'll assume a smattering of consults in there too, because you're a specialist. Your outpatient consult codes will be 99241-99245. We'll then toss in a splash of rechecks for good measure, looking at CPT® codes 99211-99215. In our earlier example, we looked only at NP office visits (E&M codes) and rechecks.

On the matrix below, I've keyed in Medicare's general fees for these procedures. Now, so you know, the basic assumptions are:

1. Medicare and Name Brand 1 Insurance (NB1) are equally split, 50/50
2. You have a normal Gaussian distribution of new patients, consults, and rechecks (Truth be told, you will probably do very few level 1 and 2 NP visits as the percent of your NP visits; NPs by definition are labor intensive.)
3. 26.67% of your office visits are considered new patients
   a. Of those NP visits, 20% are consults
4. Medicare is paying at Atlanta, region 1 reimbursement rates
5. NB1 is paying at 135% of Medicare rates
6. You work 48 weeks out of the year (4 weeks off) and see 30 patients per day, or 4.29/hour. (Watch for that .29, they're crafty suckers and usually require the most handholding.)
7. We'll assume that you are busy from day 1. Realistically, it may take you a few months before you are this busy, owing to marketing of you by the practice, current real needs of the practice (as opposed to what you were sold in the interview), and how quickly you can get on the various panels or insurance plans. You can always discount the factor back.
8. This is an annualized basis.

Based on the aforementioned assumptions, you'd expect to generate net revenues ($$$ in the door) of nearly $645,000. If your commercial payers were paying you 150% of Medicare, you might see that production number jump to nearly $687,000.

With revenues of $645,000/year, you'd be generating net revenue of nearly $2,800 per working day.

Your charges for this time period *might* be on the order of $850,000-$1,000,000 for the time period in question.

Now, this is a very simplistic case and even simpler argument. To think that from day 1 you'll see 30 patients a day is probably hard to imagine. Even more hard to imagine is that you may see 30 patients a day, every day, for 1 full year. But what this model does not take into account are the ancillary procedures that you may or may not perform during the year.

What this exercise does is enable you to begin to understand how both patient and payer mix impact your revenue and give you an idea of what you might generate purely from Medicare and commercial payers paying on the order of 135% of Medicare.

As I said, in terms of these types of models, I try to be conservative. To get an idea for yourself of how this might pan out, collect the following data from your prospective employer. They can offer it without feeling like they've given away the trade secrets.

1. How many weeks a year will I work (goes to your contract)?
2. Daily, how many patients might I see?
   a. New patients and consults?
   b. Rechecks?
3. Approximately what percentage of Medicare, on aggregate, are your commercial insurers (private payers)? For instance, 135% of Medicare. (see Exhibit 16 below - spreadsheet)

Once you have amassed these details, you should then go to the Medicare carrier's Web site for the CPT® codes mentioned and find out Medicare's rates for the procedures for the area in question where you'll live. This exercise should be fairly painless. Then multiply the reimbursement by the codes to get a basic feel for what you might generate as a first-year guy/gal in practice X. Remember, this is very basic. One cannot divine totally the revenues expected to be generated without knowing what the procedures and mix of those procedures is throughout the practice. This model cannot be foolproof as the patient mix in the practice will alter the outcome. Medicare just announced that for 2010 they will not reimburse physicians for consult codes. Other payers, at the time of this writing, continue to reimburse for consult codes.

Now, all of that said, before you look at those numbers and think that you are now the newest rainmaker to practice X, keep this in mind. Out of the revenue must come a variety of different cost components necessary to run the business. Those tidbits amalgamate to create a neat little term known as overhead, or, put simply, the cost of

**EXHIBIT 16.**

If an office based physician in Atlanta (region 1)

| | CPT Code | Fees for Medicare | Fees for Name Brand 1 | Number of patients - Medicare | Medicare Revenue | Number of patients - NB 1 | NB 1 Revenue |
|---|---|---|---|---|---|---|---|
| New patient visits | 99201 | $ 37.48 | $ 48.72 | 76.8 | $ 2,878.46 | 76.8 | $ 3,742.00 |
| | 99202 | $ 65.12 | $ 84.66 | 153.6 | $ 10,002.43 | 153.6 | $ 13,003.16 |
| | 99203 | $ 96.28 | $ 125.16 | 307.2 | $ 29,577.22 | 307.2 | $ 38,450.38 |
| | 99204 | $ 145.57 | $ 189.24 | 153.6 | $ 22,359.55 | 153.6 | $ 29,067.42 |
| | 99205 | $ 182.34 | $ 237.04 | 76.8 | $ 14,003.71 | 76.8 | $ 18,204.83 |
| consults | 99241 | $ 50.88 | $ 66.14 | 19.2 | $ 976.90 | 19.2 | $ 1,269.96 |
| | 99242 | $ 93.33 | $ 121.33 | 38.4 | $ 3,583.87 | 38.4 | $ 4,659.03 |
| | 99243 | $ 127.67 | $ 165.97 | 76.8 | $ 9,805.06 | 76.8 | $ 12,746.57 |
| | 99244 | $ 186.78 | $ 242.81 | 38.4 | $ 7,172.35 | 38.4 | $ 9,324.06 |
| | 99245 | $ 231.59 | $ 301.07 | 19.2 | $ 4,446.53 | 19.2 | $ 5,780.49 |
| Recheck visits | 99211 | $ 21.40 | $ 27.82 | 264 | $ 5,649.60 | 264 | $ 7,344.48 |
| | 99212 | $ 38.72 | $ 50.34 | 528 | $ 20,444.16 | 528 | $ 26,577.41 |
| | 99213 | $ 62.21 | $ 80.87 | 1056 | $ 65,693.76 | 1056 | $ 85,401.89 |
| | 99214 | $ 94.21 | $ 122.47 | 528 | $ 49,742.88 | 528 | $ 64,665.74 |
| | 99215 | $ 127.18 | $ 165.33 | 264 | $ 33,575.52 | 264 | $ 43,648.18 |
| | | | *Totals:* | 3600 | $ 279,912.00 | 3600 | $ 363,885.60 |

Possible Revenue: $ 643,797.60

$ 2,751.27 Per day

doing business. Think you've boned up on overhead? Don't kid yourself. There's more out there.

- What is the aggregate reimbursement of your payers relative to Medicare (eg, 175 % would be pretty phenomenal)?
- How often does the practice review contracts?

- Do you examine, either semiannually or annually, physician productivity either by RVUs or some other measure?

## OVERHEAD: THE COST TO DOING BUSINESS
## FUN/EDUCATIONAL ANECDOTE NUMBER 10

I was interviewing a young MD who was just finishing Fellowship. He was in a very demanding specialty, was very bright, and was a definite hire target. One thing I found to be interesting, though, is that when he and I dined, he told me he was excited to join our group as he thought he'd be able to reduce overhead. Now, props to the young buck for even knowing what overhead was, but there comes a line that trundles the margins where knowledge and humility meet and then, on the other side of that line, the walls of knowledge spin dismally away, dropping to a rocky floor of hubris. I suppose it's sort of akin to that fine line between genius and absolute, off-the-hook insanity. In any event, the edge is high, the fall steep, but the recovery is very doable.

## OVERHEAD: YOU KNOW IT, SO WHAT IS IT!?
## FIXED OPERATING COSTS

Your total operating costs are broadly broken down into fixed and variable costs. Fixed costs are what you might assume. They constitute the expenses that are there, regardless of whether or not you're seeing patients. They are, well, fixed. You pay them whether or not you have revenue coming into the practice. For instance, the building you either own or rent is a fixed expense. Whether or not you see patients is irrelevant. You still need to pay the fixed cost of the agreement you have regarding that building. Most employee costs are fixed, as you have to pay their salaries, regardless of whether or not they're being productive. Yet you can have some variability in there, too, for those folks who are PRN or who have flexible hours. Other fixed costs include items such as equipment, computer systems, or ultrasound machines. You pay for those, whether you use them or not.

*Variable operating costs*

Variable costs are those costs that rise or fall relative to production. They include any costs inherently tied into the product. For instance, the variable cost of a widget might be $2 where it costs a group $2 for every widget it makes. Let's say that your fixed costs are $20 to make that widget. To find out the true cost of making widgets, you'd have a simple formula of $20 (fixed costs) + $2x where $2 is your per unit variable cost and "x" is your number of units. So if you made 25 widgets, the cost would be: $20+$2(25)=$70. It costs you $70 in total costs (fixed plus variable) to make 25 widgets and so the total cost, the variability, is predicated on the number of units produced. Thus, variable costs.

See, here's the thing. Sure, you can reduce overhead, as suggested by the new MD in *Fun/Educational Anecdote Number 10*. I could have done that the next day by firing 25 staff members. The intellectual question is, really, ***how*** are you going to do that? Maybe with the primer that follows, at least you'll have an understanding of how, on the aggregate, you might play a role, either in increasing the overhead percentage or decreasing it. But in any event, don't kid yourself into thinking that you know all there is to know about overhead. Though easy in concept, it's just not that easy in application.

Overhead is the cost to run the practice, the operating costs of the practice. It is normally expressed as a percent and reflects the relationship between expenses and revenues. Generally, at least in health care, we express overhead as a percentage. For instance, if it costs you $50 to run a practice, and you generate $100 in revenue, you are running a 50% overhead ratio. That is, $50/$100 = 50%. That tells you that for every 1 dollar you bring into the practice, $.50 goes out in bills and operating costs. All in all, not too bad, depending on your specialty. That also means that there may be $50 to be distributed to the owners/partners, either in increased draw (in an LLC) or a bonus (in a professional corporation), depending on debt load and other factors.

The components for calculating overhead can vary a little bit. Remember, in general, when we look at overhead, we're looking at what it costs to run the business but also how much of the revenue is left over to go to the owners of the business. So, in our example above, we considered that $50 went to all costs and $50 then went out to the shareholders in some shape or form. That said, some practices calculate overhead using all MD compensation and benefits ("all" meaning the partners and the associate, employed physicians) while some practices remove only the owner/shareholder costs to determine overhead. The variation offers an idea of how much money is paid out to *all* physicians vs how much is available for distribution to the owners. Splitting hairs, really, but worth looking at, just the same.

If you really want to excite the group you're interviewing with, ask them their overhead percent. Nearly every practice, no matter how large or small, should have a very good grasp on that number. Then do them one better. Ask them if, in calculating their overhead percent, the employed MDs and their associated expenses fall above the line or below the line. This'll knock 'em for a loop!

Exhibit 17 displays a few things. After our trip back from LaLa Land, where you can keep costs static, we'll note the impact on our MD distributions in Year 2. As you can see, in Year 1 the practice had revenues of $2.5 million with expenses of $1.175 million for an acceptable overhead rate of 47%. You'll note that our employee costs are on the high end of the range, but in our acceptable parameters

**EXHIBIT 17.**

Cost function in Overhead:

**Version 1:**
**Year 1**

Income statement for Practice X

| | | Income |
|---|---|---|
| *Income:* | $ 2,500,000.00 | 100.00% |
| Expenses: | | |
| Employees* | $ 625,000.00 | 25.00% |
| Equipment | $ 300,000.00 | 12.00% |
| Med/mal | $ 100,000.00 | 4.00% |
| Rent/occupancy | $ 150,000.00 | 6.00% |
| *Total Expenses:* | $ 1,175,000.00 | 47.00% Overhead |
| | | |
| Distribution to partners: | $ 1,325,000.00 | |

**Version 2: Increased revenue,**
**Year 2** (v. Y 1), static costs

Income statement for Practice X

| | | Income |
|---|---|---|
| *Income:* | $ 3,000,000.00 | 100.00% |
| Expenses: | | |
| Employees* | $ 625,000.00 | 20.83% |
| Equipment | $ 300,000.00 | 10.00% |
| Med/mal | $ 100,000.00 | 3.33% |
| Rent/occupancy | $ 150,000.00 | 5.00% |
| *Total Expenses:* | $ 1,175,000.00 | 39.17% Overhead |
| | | |
| Distribution to partners: | $ 1,825,000.00 | |

Increasing revenue while keeping costs static lowered overhead v. year 1 ... 7.83% while increasing shareholder distributions.

**Version 3 Decreased revenue,**
**Year 2** (v. Y 1), static costs

Income statement for Practice X

| | | Income |
|---|---|---|
| *Income:* | $ 2,000,000.00 | 100.00% |
| Expenses: | | |
| Employees* | $ 625,000.00 | 31.25% |
| Equipment | $ 300,000.00 | 15.00% |
| Med/mal | $ 100,000.00 | 5.00% |
| Rent/occupancy | $ 150,000.00 | 7.50% |
| *Total Expenses:* | $ 1,175,000.00 | 58.75% Overhead |
| | | |
| Distribution to partners: | $ 825,000.00 | |

*Reducing* revenue while keeping costs static *increased* overhead v. year 1 ... 11.75% while reducing shareholder distributions.

just the same at 25%. Our occupancy costs are right about where we want them, too, at 6% of our revenues.

Now, look at Year 2, Version 2. Our costs stayed static (again, a brief rumble through LaLa Land) and our net revenue increased fairly significantly. That not only increased the distribution available to the shareholder MDs, it also reduced our overall overhead percentage to an exceptional 39%. More interestingly, you'll note our employee costs. In real terms, they did not drop. But as a percent of overhead, they did. Again, overhead analysis is a function of our revenue. So, the impact of increased revenue bounced against static employee costs lowers our employee piece of overhead to 20.83%. Fantastic. Now, before you go assuming that this is a shell game of some sort, a reasonable argument can be levied for the numbers presented. It would seem that, given that employee costs have remained static, you have become more efficient in your manpower allocation or used technology more appropriately, and by doing so have leveraged those resources to generate an additional $500K in revenue.

However, look what happens in Year 2, Version 3 when we've managed to keep costs static but have lost revenue. A different ball game all together. Distributions to MDs decrease, overhead percentage balloons, and our employee costs as a percent of revenues have gone off the charts. Now you could posit the converse argument (among many) that I offered in the last paragraph with regard to staff. However, since revenue generation (widget-making) is an MD function, I'd certainly start there first in my analysis of why the revenues had dropped of the precipice.

In any event, keep in mind that none of these measurements occurs in a vacuum and a variety of factors must be contemplated whilst reviewing any numbers.

Let's look at another example. As you can see, in theory, looking at overhead is pretty easy, pretty cut and dry. But, managing it, in reality, is a different animal altogether. If you cut Suzy Q, how will she feed her family? That's why I'm into running a lean machine in terms of staff; many of these folks work very hard for you and the average salary, I'd think (anecdotal, but given the nature of the business, probably not far off), is between $21,000-$40,000 per year. Depending on your area of the country, that may not translate into a lot of money left over for family discretionary spending once the bills are paid. So, your decision on how to cut overhead, the largest expense being staff, can impact lives, sometimes negatively.

Remember, in general, reimbursements are not going up, year over year. They're dropping. And Medicare, at the time of this writing, was threatening yet another cut. If your group is heavy into Medicare, you'll be heavy into a revenue drop. At some point, the lines will intersect.

## HOW TO CUT OVERHEAD: THE SWEET SCIENCE

Actually, there's nothing sweet or scientific about it, really. Just seemed like a catchy title. Pragmatically, there are 3 ways to positively impact your overhead percentage and therewith positively impact the business's revenue stream.

1. Increase revenues, keep costs static,
2. Keep revenue inflows the same and decrease costs, or (the most optimal),
3. Increase revenue and decrease costs simultaneously.

We'll also take a look at what happens with increasing costs and increasing revenues.

As a caveat, these are overly simplified examples, as you might expect. The goal here is not to slam you with data, facts, and figures, but instead to provide you with simple, easy-to-digest samples out of which you can wrestle an understanding of practice management from the ether.

**EXHIBIT 18.**

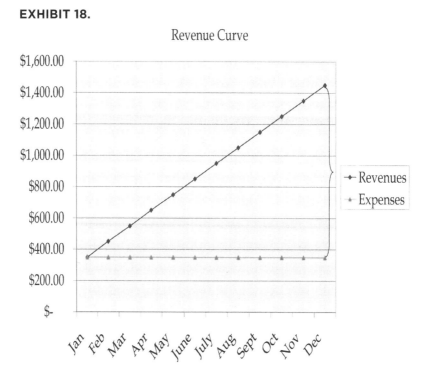

In Exhibit 18 above, you can see how a positive shift in revenue while managing costs positively impacts cash flow into the practice. The climbing dark line is incremental revenue gains added onto the previous month, while the static lighter line displays roughly the same cost per month to run the practice each month. The flat line does *not* indicate that you've only spent about $350 to run the practice. Instead, it indicates that you are spending roughly $350 each month for a total expenditure of about $4,200 for the year to run the practice. The dark line *does* show growth in revenue month over month. For instance, January showed revenue of about $350. Then, in February the practice brought in $450 or $100 more than in January. In March, the practice took in $550 or another $100 more than in February. As you can see, this graph displays, in very simple terms, how we've increased revenues and kept costs static, month over month.

That was accomplished by magic, I've no doubt, as that's what it would take to keep costs static for any period of time. Again, on this adventure to LaLa Land, we'd realize that this was virtually, nay, wholly impossible. Nonetheless, in our example, our receipts increase $100 a month more than the previous month. Our end-of-year revenues were $10,800, with a profit (total revenues minus total costs) of $6,600. This translates to a year-end overhead of 38.89% or, as you know, $0.3889 of each dollar earned going out the door to expenses. Had we run a 38.89% overhead for the year in question, we'd be overjoyed! Remember, too, the key to this exercise is not only to look at your overhead on an annual basis but to keep an eye on things on a month-to-month basis. If you did this, you'd notice that in January our overhead was 100%. Or, put a bit differently, every dollar that came in the door went out to expenses, *not including partner/shareholder salaries!* Those are extra.

In January of year X, we had expenses of $350 and revenues of $350 for a profit of $0. In February, we had expenses of $350 and revenues of $450, for a month profit of $100 and a year-to-date (YTD) profit of $100. In that case, our overhead is running about 89% YTD, but 79% for the month at hand. In March, you can see that we have a revenue of $550 and expenses of $350. A profit for the month of $200 with overhead for the month of March at 63.64%, while YTD overhead has dropped to about 78%. So, what we see is month by month our revenues are increasing and our expenses each month are about the same. We're noting a fairly significant, in terms of percentages, improvement in overhead monthly, with a slowly dropping YTD overhead.

Now, the moral to this story is: don't examine your numbers in a vacuum. You can see that we started with an astronomical overhead returning almost no money to the shareholders. But when we look at overhead, we don't want to look at it as a single point, as a single blip in the practice. Because in some months you might have more revenue coming in, whether you've worked harder, the payers have finally paid accurately, or both. In other months, you might've taken a respite in Bora Bora and/or payers were slow in paying. It's a good example of why we look at numbers and trends over time.

In Exhibit 18, the year-end overhead is a nice 38.89%, leaving a fair chunk of change to distribute to the physician-shareholders, as evidenced by the widening gap between the dark line and light line.

## CHASING YOUR TAIL — ANOTHER OVERHEAD POSSIBILITY

Another way to keep overhead in check is to keep revenue static and decrease costs. As with Exhibit 18, this is absurd. But in Exhibit 19 below, you can see that our little absurdity generated the same amount of cash each month. But our cash *position* in the practice improved dramatically, as we continuously dropped our operating costs month over month. You can see the area to the right, as noted by the bracket, growing wider, indicating, in graphical terms, an increase in revenue over expenses as the year progresses.

You might have surmised that these graphical depictions are fairly off the wall. Sure, that's true. If you didn't notice this, then we need to talk. What you should get from this review is a good understanding of the relationship between revenues and expenses and how those are inextricably woven into the fabric of any business in or outside of health care. As you might imagine, it is probably nearly impossible to keep

**EXHIBIT 19.**

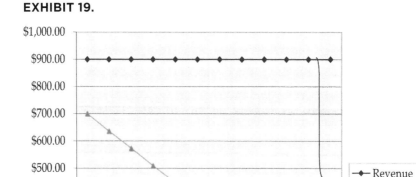

revenue or expenses static in absolute terms, for a variety of reasons, the least of which is the fact that there are 25 gazillion variables in health care operating at any given time and oftentimes they are mutually exclusive.

*And yet a third option: the BEST!*

So we've seen that either holding costs static and increasing revenues or keeping revenues static and decreasing costs are keys to widening the profitability margin. Now the third, and obviously best option, is to increase revenues *while* decreasing costs. As you can see from Exhibit 20, our profitability increases rapidly in this model. We are increasing, month over month, our revenues by $100 while cutting costs. Though this allows for a year-end overhead rate similar to our previous graphs at year's end, if things remained static, our margins would continue to improve over time.

The problem here? There's just about, as we discussed before, no way on earth that you will continue to decrease, in real terms, the costs of running your business on an ongoing basis. You can only cut so far, and even if you kept cutting, there would come a day of reckoning where you realize a factual cut. Eventually you hit rock bottom. After all, you can only fire so many staff members, you can only get *out* of so many leases, you can only run with no new equipment for so long. That's where you're getting to, after a while.

**EXHIBIT 20.**

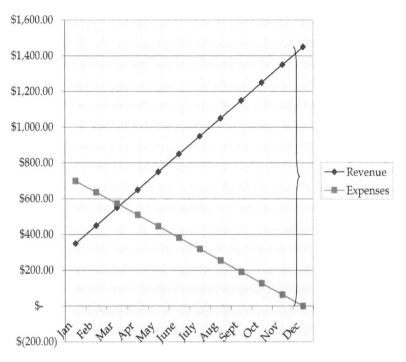

## THE BENEFITS OF CONTROLLING COSTS

Exhibit 21 is our train wreck. It is closer to a more realistic depiction of what one might actually see in a group practice, apropos of costs. But I hope you never experience this cost issue to this extreme. I would not expect the continuation of the problems displayed in this graph, given good, sound management and physician involvement.

What you see here is a good start to the year. This graph shows an overhead rate of 29% in January. We enjoyed revenues of $350 with expenses of $100 ($100/$350 = 28.57% overhead). But the overhead rate in February jumps to 61% for the month ($450 in revenue, $275 in expenses; $275/$450 = 61.11%), meaning, as we've discussed, that $0.61 of each dollar in the door is going out the door in expenses. No need to worry just yet, but definitely something to be privy to and it's time for management to begin asking some fairly robust questions. In March, you can see the light expense line moving closer and closer to the revenue line. Overhead for the month is a little lofty, at about 68%, but nothing to drive you to drink. Then in April you see the cost line crossing the revenue line. For that month, we're running more than 100% overhead, meaning we're spending more than we're bringing in. A little scary. For the month, this is a mess and requires immediate attention. If you looked at this over time, you'd note too that overhead has crept to a YTD rate of 76% (most groups, depending on specialty, will run overhead of ~50%-55%). Something has to give and the ship is not turning around.

What you see graphically depicted is the problem of too much spending and not enough revenue to cover the costs. The revenue is increasing, but the expenditures are outpacing, or nearly outpacing, all revenue gains. There are any number of reasons why our Graph 4 group is getting ready for a big hurt, but some problems could be variable costs that are getting out of hand, physicians not seeing enough patients, or all of the above.

Where you see the expense line cross the revenue line, you know for that month that the group spent more than what came in. In a month, that might not be fatal. Over time, well . . . remember that adage I threw out about it costing $10 to make a chair, you'd sell it for $9, and make up the difference on volume? That's what they're looking at. Remember, no matter how many chairs you make at $10, selling them for $9 you will never cover your costs.

At year's end, the group in question has run a 101.25% overhead, meaning, basically, that the group is borrowing to get by. Not a good spot to be in. In this case, Awesome the administrator has just morphed into Awful the administrator, even if the issue was not his or her fault.

This graph shows, too, that we are not gaining any ground when our costs rise in concert with our revenues. In other words, you are probably working harder and faster but your rising costs (as evidenced by the increased revenues) are eating up any gains in the margin.

In any event, as with any business, the cost to run a practice will, over time, increase, whether by design or covert creep. The key is to manage the creep, control it, and try to mitigate it via increased revenues and cost containment.

## DECISIONS, DECISIONS

Above we chatted ever so briefly about the ramifications of costs. Remember, just about every decision you and yours make apropos of the running of the practice will impact, in one way or another, costs. For instance, Dr Mendit wants a new technician, that adds, say $30,000 to the salary costs, exclusive of the 25% or so in added benefits, etc. So, adding Tech 1 costs Dr Mendit roughly $37,500 annually. Remember, too, that Tech 1 will probably want and/or expect a raise next year based on merit or a cost of living (COL) increase. COL is going to run you nearly 3% annually, which means Tech 1 then moves to about $38,625 in salary and benefits in Year 2. Now, the question becomes, will you generate $37,500 in revenue by having Tech 1 on board, or is she there just to appease and make life easier for Dr. Mendit? This is an essential question because, as an administrator, I could hang my hat and make an argument for the added FTE on

**EXHIBIT 21.**

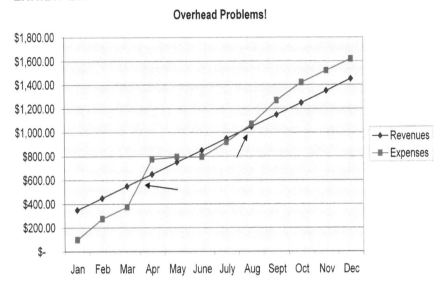

the latter choice (generating revenue), but the former does nothing for me and as the arbiter for the practice's best interest (eg, all partner owners *equally*), I don't know that hiring Tech 1 makes sense. It might make sense if the group shared expenses based on some sort of consumption formula, but if this is an added cost to all MDs just to improve Dr Mendit's life, I'm thinking I might shoot that down. Let's take a surreal, otherworldly look:

*Pre-Tech 1*

Revenue:     $100
Expenses:    $50
Overhead:     50% ($50/$100 = $50, roughly goes back to the partners)

*Adding Suzy Q - Post-Tech 1*

Revenue:     $100
Expenses:    $51
Overhead:     51% ($51/$100 = roughly $49 goes back to partners)
So, with these fictional figures, Suzy Q did nothing to impact my revenue, and yet adding Suzy Q negatively impacts the MDs on the whole while positively helping Dr Mendit and his quality of life.

Bottom line, all decisions have an impact, large or small. And each decision should be analyzed in the scheme of what the partners are comfortable with and what is best for the business.

## AND YET, MORE

Normally, as we've said, overhead is expressed as a percent. You might have a practice that runs a 50% overhead, meaning if you have revenues of $100, $50 gets paid out to cover the expenses of running the practice (staff salaries, rent, equipment leases, meds and supplies, med/mal) while the remaining $50 may get paid out to the physician-owners of the group. (Remember, you can look at employed physicians as a cost to the practice. When you become a partner, I'd then pull you out of the formula and drop you below the line.)

Another way to examine this is if you were a partner and you wanted to earn $500,000 each year and you knew the practice ran about 50% overhead, you know you'd need to produce (not in charges but in actual receipts: dollars in the door) somewhere north of $1,000,000 in revenue per year. Though attainable in many specialties, you need to be burning it down* to generate that kind of money. (*Author's note: definitionally, "burning it down" can loosely be translated as equal to minimal family time and minimal vacation + maximum work time and maximum patient encounters.)

*Above the line, below the line*

Just when you thought we'd beaten this thing into the ground, we'll dig a bit further. Some groups will lump in associate MDs *and* owners to see how many of the total dollars in the door go to physician pay. Others separate out the owners and keep the employee MDs in as a cost.

This isn't rocket science. But, apropos of overhead, it gives you a different method for looking at how the cash that flows in gets distributed to physicians. Again, if I'm looking at these figures purely for the Partners, I'd review relative to revenues that get disbursed to the owner-physicians. After all, when all is said and done, they are the ones who own the business. But another method of looking at this is how much money that flows in is distributable to *all* physicians. Exhibit 22 is an example.

So, overhead, *including employed MDs as a cost,* is 47% (in Version 1 above). Now, let's drop employed MD costs below the line, or after net revenues have been calculated. We'll say that pulling out employed MD salary and benefits reduces employee costs by $200,000. In Version 2 above, our employee costs dropped from $625,000 to $425,000.

As you can see in our example, overhead dropped to 39% when we pulled out employed MDs. What does this mean to us, practically speaking? Well, it offers you a measure of how much money is being parsed out to *all* MDs vs just the partner MDs, indicating that, for one thing, the practice is running at a fairly efficient clip.

**EXHIBIT 22.**

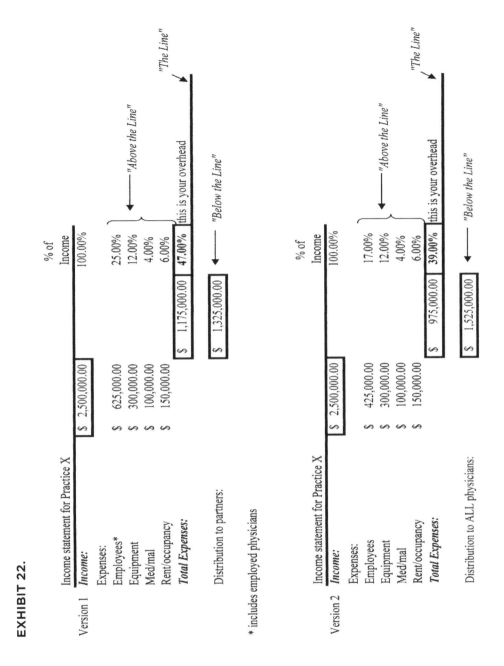

Version 1

Income statement for Practice X

| | | | % of Income |
|---|---|---|---|
| **Income:** | $ | 2,500,000.00 | 100.00% |
| Expenses: | | | |
| Employees* | $ | 625,000.00 | 25.00% |
| Equipment | $ | 300,000.00 | 12.00% |
| Med/mal | $ | 100,000.00 | 4.00% |
| Rent/occupancy | $ | 150,000.00 | 6.00% |
| **Total Expenses:** | $ | 1,175,000.00 | **47.00%** |

this is your overhead

Distribution to partners: $ 1,325,000.00

"Above the Line"

"The Line"

"Below the Line"

* includes employed physicians

Version 2

Income statement for Practice X

| | | | % of Income |
|---|---|---|---|
| **Income:** | $ | 2,500,000.00 | 100.00% |
| Expenses: | | | |
| Employees | $ | 425,000.00 | 17.00% |
| Equipment | $ | 300,000.00 | 12.00% |
| Med/mal | $ | 100,000.00 | 4.00% |
| Rent/occupancy | $ | 150,000.00 | 6.00% |
| **Total Expenses:** | $ | 975,000.00 | **39.00%** |

this is your overhead

Distribution to ALL physicians: $ 1,525,000.00

"Above the Line"

"The Line"

"Below the Line"

This is an individual consideration and one that each group must determine. The key is defining the measurement tool and then sticking with it. This will enable you to look at your costs and overhead on a year-by-year basis with consistency. This assures the group that they will perform an apples-to-apples look and, when the definition is hammered out, enables the MDs and management staff to look very closely at deviations from expected overhead percentages.

*Costs*

Generally speaking, your 3 largest cost components in a privately held medical practice will be staff (with benefits, usually 20%-27% of net revenue or dollars in the door), rent expense (depending on whether buildings are owned or not, generally 5%-7% of revenue), and your equipment costs (depending in your practice specialty type, eg, cardiology with lots of capital costs or internal medicine with relatively few). So, again, with our round figures, let's look at the breakdown:

Charges:                          $175
Revenues:                        $100  (these are NET of charges; actual collected money)
Staff salaries and benefits:  $24
Equipment:                        $7  (we're in a capital-intensive specialty)
Rent:                                 $6
Other:                                $6  (med supplies, med/mal, travel, IT, other)
Net revenue:                     $57

Two ways to look at this are that our overhead is 43% ($43/$100) or that $57 (net revenue, what's left over after expenses) now gets split out to the physician-owners. To carry it further, let's say that we have 10 MD owners (just to keep things nice, tidy, and round) and our 10 MD owners are equal share owners. That is, their compensation (depending on your tax status) is what's left over and they each split the net revenues equally. So our MD partners would receive $5.70 each in salary ($57/10).

Do not get overly hooked on the overhead percentages. Many young docs enter the interview process asking the very legitimate question of "What's your overhead?" It's good that so many physicians are beginning to get a feel for that question. But there's another component that you must be aware of and one to consider when evaluating a practice.

## PROPS TO THE HIGH OVERHEAD GROUP

Group X generates revenue as modeled above. Group Y is investing heavily in an information technology/CT hybrid that produces 3D diagnostic images, loads them directly onto any PC in the world, and is approved by Medicare and reimbursable. Now, Group Y has bought the new Gig-a-ma-kallit and has jumped through all appropriate hoops related to the Gig-a-ma-kallit. They've spoken with their administrator, or run out that the product is clinically efficacious and reimbursable. They've consulted with their attorneys (where necessary) to structure a deal and they've spoken with their accountants about the Section 179 accelerated depreciation for the unit.

The group has determined that their current overhead is right at about 43%, just like Group X above. But Group Y has now hunkered down for an overhead soon to be 90%-based on the acquisition of the Gig-a-ma-kallit. The groups are similarly situated, both in geography (East coast), specialty, and general reimbursement pattern. But the shareholder MDs stand to make **more money** from the new procedure, even given the increased operating costs, and are all for it. How is that possible, you ask, at a 90% overhead rate? Here's how:

**EXHIBIT 23.**

Props to the High Overhead Group?

**Group X**

| Charges: | $ 175.00 | | |
|---|---|---|---|
| Revenues: | $ 100.00 | | (these are NET of charges; actual collected money) |
| Staff Expenses: | | $ 24.00 | |
| Equipment: | | $ 7.00 | $7 (we're in a capital intensive specialty) |
| Rent: | | $ 6.00 | |
| Other: | | $ 6.00 | (med supplies, med/mal, travel, IT, other) |
| *Total Expenses:* | | $ 43.00 | |
| Net Revenue: | | $ 57.00 | |
| Overhead: | | 43.00% | |
| Distribution to each of 10 partners: | | $ 5.70 | (Net revenue/10 partners) |

**Group Y**

| Charges: | $ 1,050.00 | | (with Giga installed) |
|---|---|---|---|
| Revenues: | $ 600.00 | | (net collected money) |
| Staff Expenses: | | $ 25.00 | (slight increase in staff cost due to Giga) |
| Equipment: | | $ 500.00 | (major increase in equipment costs associated with current equipment plus the Giga) |
| Rent: | | $ 6.00 | |
| Other: | | $ 9.00 | (slight increase due to Giga) |
| *Total Expenses:* | | $ 540.00 | |
| Net Revenue: | | $ 60.00 | |
| Overhead: | | 90.00% | |
| Distribution to each of 10 partners: | | $ 6.00 | (Net revenue/10 partners) |

| | | |
|---|---|---|
| Increase in Overhead: | 1256% | |
| Increase in Revenue: | 600% | |
| Increase in sharholder revenue: | 5.26% | |
| "Real" increase in overhead cost: | $ 497.00 | |

With the original 10 partners in Group Y, you can see that the shareholder MDs' compensation has now jumped from $5.70/MD to $6.00/MD ($60/10 vs $57/10MDs). This is an increase of 5.264% in physician/shareholder compensation while increasing overhead about 1.256% or $497.

Now, is this an absurd model? You tell me. The purpose, though, is to show that sometimes even a high overhead group can generate revenue and displays that the added overhead, the added expenditure, can be worth the investment. The key rests in the physician owners' philosophy, generally, toward overhead, shareholder value, and the risk of embracing new and expensive technology that may or may not be around for a number of years.

## THAT'S ALL FOLKS . . .

Like I said, I like when new physicians come in for an interview and tell me how they're going to "lower your overhead." To wit, I like to ask "How?"

The economics of the health care model, really, most business models, is that you either see more patients (or, in business, make and sell more widgets) and provide good care (make a good product) or you don't. But just wanting to make more money will not meet either of these 2 requirements.

Here's the thing. The overhead proposition is fairly simple in theory, but not so much in practice. Its function in a practice is as individual as each physician. To presume in an interview that you understand all of the component parts of a practice's overhead is an oversimplification on an easy theory but fairly complicated model.

## *Miscellaneous Ramblings and Assorted Other Thoughts*

### TO ELECTRONIC MEDICAL RECORD (EMR) OR NOT TO EMR & IT

Trite title, right? Ok. Point stipulated. But as trite as it is, that is a question (or statement) that will be pondered by many, if not all, medical groups over the next 2-10 years. Now, this book is neither dedicated to EMRs nor trying to make a point either way, but I could easily write a full book on the ups and downs alone, the trials and tribulations, of looking for, installing, and living with an EMR. But I would like to touch on some of the points here that I think will be of value to you as you look at practices and their data management, how much they're on the forefront of technology, and so on.

Just so you know, I'm a big fan, and big isn't adjective enough to handle my love of EMRs. Now, tempering that against the intricacies, product obsolescence (whether planned or happenstance), and cost overruns, I still love EMRs. There are a variety of reasons, but let me toss out a few that come to mind.

EMRs go by a variety of acronyms but mean, essentially, the same thing. The patient's medical record is stored and moved around (the office, etc) electronically. The EMR is a full rendering of the medical record, from notes, dictations, and scrips to diagnosis, charting of values, etc. A fully integrated EMR, as I define for the purposes of this book, is an EMR that is tied in, integrated, with a practice management system.

This seamlessness, in my experience, leaves very little room for error, as the record and its related billing data passes on to the billing and practice management components of the computer system without intervention or special interface programming. It is seamless to the user. There are many EMRs out there that do not integrate in this manner or can have integration code written so that the EMR "talks" with the current (or new) practice management system. But those come with some cost.

EMRs come in a variety of shapes and sizes, expenses, and functional realms. The right one can make a practitioner's job a dream, or at worst, bearable. The wrong one can make a difficult job that much more so.

EMRs can also yield a tremendous amount of valuable data regarding the practice. Aside from the reporting of the practice management software, the EMR can offer you a look at how your group is treating certain disease states and would enable a group to analyze its treatment patterns, by MD or clinician, against nationally set standards from the various societies. This data can be boiled down to make clinical improvement and assist in closing that clinical care loop I mentioned earlier. It can help you assure that you are treating all of your patients as best as possible given current clinical norms and protocols.

Also, being in control of your data, especially during this time of quality medicine, enables you to bargain from a position of strength. You'll be able to demonstrate to payers that you are in control of your outcomes, you understand them, and you are practicing good quality care. As of this writing, there aren't a lot of private practices throughout the country who are doing this on an ongoing basis. By the time this goes to print, that may have changed.

What EMRs can offer is valuable to clinicians, too. EMRs can assist in the clinical decision making process, can track meds and missed scrips, can monitor missed appointments, and assist in assuring that proper follow-up and closure of the care loop is offered.

How? For one thing, you can, on some EMRs, integrate clinical documents from your governing specialty association, which will help you to validate your care decisions and provide, based on updated documentation, the most recent thoughts regarding the level of care for your patients. For instance, the Grand Mall Association might have a solid peer-reviewed document issued that states "patients with XXYYZZ Syndrome should have their toes flagellated every 6 months and a simultaneous echocardiogram performed to gauge level of heart function during flagellation." In some EMR systems, you can program these components into the software, so that when a patient presents with XXYYZZ Syndrome, a flag pops up on the system and alerts you to consider flagellation coupled with an echo. Be advised, this approach does NOT take the decision making out of the clinician's hands. Instead, it offers the clinician tools to better manage the patient's care based on the most recent guidelines available. It offers a bit of redundancy, if you will, a backstop to assist the clinician.

The next point is that an EMR can increase revenue into the practice as it assures you are ordering appropriate, clinically necessary document-based tests and studies. It seems to me that this is a twofold advantage: it increases revenues and does so by helping physicians provide optimal patient care.

EMRs also close, what I like to call, the clinical care loop. As busy as practitioners are these days, with as many patients as they see on a given day, an EMR can assist you in assuring that you are following the patient from start to finish. For instance, you may order lab tests on Patient X. You can, in some programs, order the tests from point of care and then see them the next day, inserted behind the scenes into the patient's chart. You can have an RN or skilled extender (PA, NP) review the results the next day, and if s/he sees an anomaly, they can contact the physician and alert him or her.

Additionally, EMRs assist in closing the clinical care loop, as they can be built to assure that follow-up appointments are contemplated by the physician and ordered on the system. You can easily validate that patients follow-up on their orders so that they return for needed care. This ensures that patients do not fall through the cracks, offering good, or at least clinically sound care, while helping to mitigate some medical malpractice exposure. How? Well, if you've ordered Patient X to return in 6 months for a pacemaker follow-up, you obviously have concern that Patient X needs constant follow-up for his pacer. If he misses the appointment, how can you prove that you followed up with him on his follow-up care? You can check to see that the order was issued, that Patient X was notified in writing (electronic letter in his chart), and maybe a call was made to his house and documented in the chart. Is this foolproof? Of course not. Nothing in life is absolute. But it is cleaner, and systems can be automated to the point of assisting as much as is possible in patient care and communication.

EMRs with practice management (PM) systems can also assist you in your billing. Many have a built in "scrubber" of sorts, which looks at what you've done in the patient exam and lets you know what CPT® code the exam might warrant. Remember, this is only the system's "thought" based on what it knows or has been programmed with. The ultimate decision, and the documentation to back up the claim, is always predicated on the practitioner. But many EMRs will "read" your inputs and let you know that you have performed enough components to bill a level 4 office visit, for instance. (That said, I'd always recommend internal coding audits to assure that you are not upcoding, that care is coded appropriately, and that codes used make sense. EMRs are neither foolproof nor infallible.)

Also, after the claims have been coded out, many "scrubbers" will look the claims over for conflicts of diagnosis and CPT® codes. They may do this by looking at Correct Coding Initiative (CCI) edits which are offered by Medicare and essentially tells you what can and cannot be coded together. Why does this help? Many e-filing systems go through clearing houses. The claim might be submitted from your system, to the clearing house, and then on to the payer. The claim might be scrubbed at the clearing house level. If you have some claims that fail edit, they'll turn around to you overnight to be investigated and corrected, then resubmitted. This is important, because if claims went on to Private Payer 1, and the claims did not match, they might be adjudicated, taking 15-30 days, and would then be denied. You would then need to research the claims and refile. So you can see you've avoided the pain of waiting for the adjudication.

Medicine is moving at the speed of light. But clinical embracing of IT and its associated infrastructure is not moving in kind. The reason? Well, in part due to the cost. The IT infrastructure and its components are expensive and can initially slow clinicians down. But once implemented, many of these tools provide immeasurable benefit. With options like "carry forward" of the last note and updating much of the preloading of info can be accomplished with these tools. However, clinicians would be wise to remember that even if data is carried forward from a previous visit, it is incumbent upon the physician to *always* assure that the patient information is accurate, up to date, and timely. That is, clinicians should *never* wholly rely on data that has been carried forward, as conditions and the patient's status are sure to have changed. EMRs may bring the data forward as a time saver, but clinicians must then review each item carefully and thoroughly to assure that the new visit is documented appropriately.

Also, data is becoming the key. How you store it, manage it, and use it. There are programs out there that can help you review your data. What I liked to do was use association-derived, nationally accepted guidelines to examine my data vs what was out there nationally.

For instance, how we were treating condition X relative to our national association's criteria. Did we treat X appropriately in 90% of the cases, as indicated? If not, were there contraindications for that treatment modality? The reason this is becoming key is that the specter of "pay for performance" is rearing its ugly head. Now, in theory, paying for performance, that is, paying for good, sound, and basic outcomes makes sense. But, the hobgoblin to the theory is practice. Who determines quality? And who determines what good quality care is? My personal concern is that if this is not addressed by the various associations throughout medicine, establishing some basic quality measures, the government will step in and tell MDs what quality is. And we know how good the government is at doing things it has no idea about. Do you want someone in Washington telling you what good medicine is? And yet Medicare, in 2007, offered an incentive to physicians via its Physician Quality Reporting Initiative (PQRI) which now is optional and will, in the future, be required to maintain a certain level of reimbursement from Medicare. Does Medicare know quality? With due respect to Medicare and the fine folks who work there and work very hard, I'd suggest not really.

Many EMRs also can have interfaces written so that many of your diagnostic imaging tools can seamlessly meld with the patient's record. Interfaces are programs written so one computer with one program on it can talk with another computer that operates a different program. When implemented, they should operate transparently within the EMR platform. So, accessing an ultrasound can be done seamlessly within the patient's chart instead of popping in and out of multiple screens at the point of care.

There are also, or can be, cost savings. Once fully EMRed, you can review patient charts for additional savings or run data for new modalities (some practice management packages will allow this). That is, if the new Gig-a-ma-kallit mentioned earlier is available, how do you know if there might be a demand? Well, you can look to your own patient database to see if some patients meet those criteria. You can mine that data, issue a flier or direct mail piece, and then man the phones.

EMRs are usually built such that you can reduce your transcription expense. Here's how it might work. You see the patient and check boxes on the intake component. That piece loads certain vignettes into the record which can eliminate virtually all of the transcription. You will then probably need to dictate, either via digital service or a voice recognition software, the impression and plan.

Another neat option is the ability to access your system from anywhere in the world. That may be as close as your bedroom when you're on call or in Khodzhent, Tajikistan, if you're so inclined. As long as you can get onto the internet, which obviously means that as long as you have access, you can work out a secure connection to your charts.

Remember, it's all about the data, and control and management of the data. Vis-à-vis contracting, many times in health care, contracting payers rely on the fact that the physicians don't have good data. So the payers may, just may, try to run the MDs over during contracting. The better your data, the better you (and your colleagues) understand it, the more power you have. And you truly have power with your data.

Another benefit is better management of the AR component. Many integrated EMRs offer the option to work accounts by payer, meaning if Private Payer 1 is not paying on a timely basis, you'll have the data at your fingertips and you can identify why that might be. Maybe it's an office visit on every patient. Maybe it's a particular drug or diagnostic test. In the old days, it would take days, maybe months, to figure out what was going on and why. At that point, your fun-loving commercial payer had moved on to the next hot idea designed to slow down payments to you.

I've been involved with a few rather bad computer installations and I've been party to a few very good installations and, from an administrator's point of view, the good are far more fun than the bad.

So, regarding your new group, are they looking at an EMR? Are they thinking of an EMR? Are they looking at some hybrid thereof using, maybe, a document storage/management facility and image-sharing from their imaging modalities? If they have an EMR, how do they use the data they are aggregating?

IT infrastructure is essential. Are they planning? Remember, with an IT infrastructure comes new workload. While your administrator should have a good feel for the system and its requirements, depending on how robust your system is and how many MDs in the group, you might consider farming out the IT component.

Do they have or need an IT infrastructure? If the group you're joining has an IT infrastructure in place, do they feel they've gained from its implementation? If so, how would the MDs, and the administrative staff, either qualify or quantify that fact? There are benchmarks that could be divined, such as increased patient flow, better management of patient care, better cash flow due to better patient management, better care (using clinical guidelines), and better management of your accounts receivable.

## A WORD ABOUT ROIs

Many projects entered into can have a return on investment (ROI) produced to offer the shareholders an idea of what their return (financial) on their investment (purchasing a component) was.

When you look at EMRs or computer systems, for that matter, it is often very difficult to quantify the absolute savings that will come with the implementation of the EMR. For instance, you should be able to state that transcription costs can be reduced because much is auto-populated in the record. But are there added costs of having scanners in place?

Gains should be looked at in terms of increased revenue via better cash management, better and more efficient scheduling, etc.

*EMR—the emotional side*

Practice administrators are constantly in search of ways to decrease costs and, where we can, help increase revenues, whether it's through new and efficacious modalities or increased patient flow efficiencies.

As was mentioned earlier in ***Overhead***, we learned that staff costs can range from 20%-27% of your revenues. Again, that means for every dollar in the door, 0.20-0.27 cents goes back out in employee costs. Remember, employee costs are one of your biggest outlays.

What you'll be told when looking at an EMR is that you can cut down on FTE employees if you install an EMR. That may be true. But if Suzy Q Transcriptionist has been with the group for 20 years, it's not all about (or at least it shouldn't be) firing her over technology. It can be a struggle, so these decisions are not necessarily so easily made.

When I look at EMRs, I try to look at how we might gain in revenues vs offsetting by getting rid of folks. It's easier to do.

Oftentimes, too, there's a decided disconnect between the sales team and the EMR install teams. They do different jobs. From time to time, situations exist where the sales team oversells, forcing the implementation team to under deliver. What does that mean? It means that in many cases, the sales team has never set foot in a clinical setting aside from walking through the waiting room and trying to make a sale. Have they gained from their implementation? If so, can they quantify those gains, that ROI?

*Quality*

I've long been a believer that, in the delivery of medicine, good quality, and good customer service prevail. The rest will take care of itself. For instance, you might be the best orthopedic surgeon on the world. But if you act like your patients' time does not matter, you might as well have graduated from the Medical School of the Lower Aleutian Islands, South Campus. Because for all of your training, all of your hard work, you might as well have played Wiffle Ball through med school. Even though patients are now educating themselves regarding their conditions, most of their perception of quality is derived not from where you went to med school and your perceptions of self, but how they are treated, how you make them feel, *and* outcomes. If/where there is choice, they'll vote with their feet. And remember this, because it's key; patients are not singular entities. No. They are husbands, wives, sons, daughters, grandmothers, and grandfathers. So if you irritate one person, you've irritated 5 or 10 people. And, it's not just you they'll think of. It's Orthopedic Group X (of which we'll assume you're a part). So now you've not only drained the well for yourself, but you've drained it for your colleagues, too.

## MONTHLY NUMBERS

Measuring what you do offers you a variety of educational opportunities. It's what any good business does. You need to know where you were, where you are, to know where you're going. All businesses, big and small, need productivity reporting to determine what's going on and to help direct change. We noticed this in looking at overhead graphs and in our quasi-modeling of production by CPT® code by Medicare and commercial payers. All of these reports should work in concert to aid management and physicians in decision making. They are fairly critical. For instance, we looked at NB1 and NB2 as measured against Medicare. And what the data told us is that it might be time to renegotiate that contract. Now we'll take it one step further by ratcheting up a notch our look at the data available.

When I look at data, I like to look at it by physician by selected category, for the current month, deviations in the current month from the prior year (eg, June 2009 measured against June 2008), and YTD for both periods. This enables me to notice semigranular changes in the months and also ongoing changes during the course of the year, such as January to June data. Looking at the data for a period of time obviously offers you a better picture of what's going on over time, allowing the data to flatten out and normalize over a longer period of time vs the peaks, valleys, and anomalies the group might experience during 1 month's measured data.

I'm a big fan of reporting and monitoring reports. We spoke about overhead and what that means, but there should be a monthly accounting offering MDs some idea of where they, and the practice, stand. I tend to be a numbers pack rat. I'll keep data back as long and as far as I can, because it enables me to run apples-to-apples comparisons, assuring the data and its associated results have relevance. The beautiful thing about the data is that it enables you to see where you were, where you are, and helps you plot out where you want to be. If you wanted to increase revenues and you have room in your schedules, you might want to add a few patient slots. How many patients you are seeing may indicate which clinician has more room in the schedule.

Numbers are also valuable because, taken in multiple slices, that is, multiple inputs, you can get a robust view of the practice's health.

Let's dissect the graphic below. We've taken a snapshot of Dr 1 and 2s' practice for a 6-month interval. We're looking at June of the current year vs June of last year. Additionally, we'll look at the YTD up to and including June vs YTD to the same time period, through June of the prior year.

The owners of Drs 1 and 2, PC have identified the criteria in the report as keys to their success. They include a measurement of revenue collected, expenses, the overhead percent, the number of new patients each clinician sees, the number of surgeries Dr 3 performs, the RVUw of the practice (remember, relative value unit - work), and the days outstanding in AR. These, to the group, have been defined as key drivers to the organization. Other groups might, for instance, measure the number of diagnostic tests they've run or the number of rechecks ordered.

When the MDs review these numbers, they've decided to include Dr 3 in the process, even though he is employed and not yet a partner. Some groups will include associates in the review of the numbers and some will not. You would be wise to query your future employers to divine their taste for sharing data and other numerical information.

As the group examines the data with Awesome the administrator, they begin by reviewing the most current month's data and the associated YTD data. They review from left to right, examining the percent changes and the real change; that is, the dollar-value change. They compare the months (June vs June) and the YTD. The reason for examining the real numerical data is that percent changes only paint a portion of

**EXHIBIT 24.**

Drs. 1 and 2, P.C.  Practice Snapshot

Month: **JUNE**

| | 2009 Monthly | Year to Date | 2008 PY Month | PYTD | Monthly % change | Monthly real $$$ change | YTD % change | YTD real $$$ change |
|---|---|---|---|---|---|---|---|---|
| **Revenue** | | | | | | | | |
| Dr. 1 | $ 100,000.00 | $ 600,000.00 | $ 95,000.00 | $ 600,000.00 | 5.3% | $ 5,000.00 | 0.0% | $ - |
| Dr. 2 | $ 120,000.00 | $ 650,000.00 | $ 120,000.00 | $ 600,000.00 | 0.0% | $ - | 8.3% | $ 50,000.00 |
| Dr. 3 | $ 175,000.00 | $ 725,000.00 | $ 225,000.00 | $ 625,000.00 | -22.2% | $ (50,000.00) | 16.0% | $ 100,000.00 |
| *Total:* | *$ 395,000.00* | *$ 1,975,000.00* | *$ 440,000.00* | *$ 1,825,000.00* | *-10.2%* | *$ (45,000.00)* | *8.2%* | *$ 150,000.00* |
| Expenses | $ 200,000.00 | $ 950,000.00 | $ 210,000.00 | $ 1,000,000.00 | -4.8% | $ (10,000.00) | -5.0% | $ (50,000.00) |
| Overhead | 50.63% | 48.10% | 47.73% | 54.79% | | | | |
| **New Patients** | | | | | | | | |
| Dr. 1 | 20 | 120 | 18 | 120 | 11.1% | 2 | 0.0% | 0 |
| Dr. 2 | 25 | 130 | 25 | 130 | 0.0% | 0 | 0.0% | 0 |
| Dr. 3 | 30 | 145 | 40 | 130 | -25.0% | (10) | 11.5% | 15 |
| *Total:* | *75* | *395* | *83* | *380* | *-9.6%* | *(8)* | *3.9%* | *15* |
| **Surgeries** | | | | | | | | |
| Dr. 3 | 30.00 | 145.00 | 40.00 | 130.00 | -25.00% | -10 | 11.54% | 15 |
| Practice RVUw | 1750.00 | 15250.00 | 1800.00 | 14200.00 | -2.78% | -50 | 7.39% | 1050 |
| Days in AR | | 35.00 | 45.00 | | -22.22% | | | -10 |

the picture. For instance, if revenues dropped from $100 to $50 in a month, you'd have a 50% drop in revenues. This equates to a loss of $50, but is that fatal to the business? Knowing the real measurement can add another layer to the picture.

As they review the numbers, the physicians note a net overall $45,000 drop in revenue for June of 2009 vs June of 2008. This concerns them a bit, with the drop ($50,000) being attributed to Dr 3's revenue. What questions does this bring to mind? Well, maybe Dr 3 had some vacation time in early June and did not produce much. Maybe in June of last year he knocked the ball out of the park, which might've been an anomaly. Looking further, you can see that Dr 3 has had a very good year with his YTD revenue numbers up 16% or $100,000. It also seems that his revenue increase has spurred 2/3s of the growth in net revenues for the entire business, YTD. So maybe the group can cut him some slack for his current June numbers. YTD, the group is up 8.2% in revenue. As long as expenses didn't grow at a similar real rate, then the group should ostensibly be in healthier financial shape than it was in 2008.

Next, the group moved down to overhead. We note that expenses dropped $10,000 June vs June (from $210K to $200K) and YTD they are down $50,000 or 5%. What this tells us is that we seem to have been cutting costs for the first 5 months of the year, since we obviously did not save $50K in the month of June. Is Awesome the administrator better utilizing staff? Has he implemented some sort of program to better manage medical supplies, thereby showing these great savings? Have we utilized some new computer program that makes our office more efficient and has enabled us to "staff adjust"? ("Staff adjust" meaning fire someone.)

When we look at overhead as a percent, as we've discussed earlier, we note that in June of this year our overhead percent was a touch higher than in June of 2008. How is this possible? Remember, the overhead percent is a ratio of expenses to revenues. And as we discussed in the prior paragraphs, your revenues in June dropped a bit. Although your June overhead ratio is a bit higher than you like, you note that the YTD is in pretty good shape, dropping significantly vs YTD at the same time last year.

The MDs and Awesome then dropped down to new patients. You can see that new patients for Dr 3 had dropped, June vs June, but the group remained 3.9% higher in YTD new patients vs prior YTD. And, you might tie back Dr 3's drop in revenues for June with a drop in new patients. Maybe he did go on that vacation after all. The good news, again, is that we might be down in June for new patients but we're up YTD.

As they look at new patients, the group ponders organic growth. By that, I mean new patients who are not dissipated by a new MD. In other words, if I see 100 new patients with 2 clinicians, and each clinician sees 50 new patients, if I add an MD and add 10 new patients, we've seen NP growth, but have we seen what we want in growth? We now have 3 MDs seeing 110 patients, or an average of 36.67 new patients per MD. Is that good? It depends on how you look at it. But I'd like to see some significant growth in new patients visits over time if I add a clinician, because ostensibly, you've added an MD because you need more physician capacity and you're not meeting the new patient demands. Again, a matter that has some subjectivity, because maybe you've added an MD for a change in the senior doc's lifestyle.

The last few categories the group examines are Dr 3's surgeries. Again, for the month of June, he was down a bit. But YTD he is up nearly 12%. Not bad.

**EXHIBIT 25.**

Drs. 1 and 2, P.C.  Practice Snapshot

| | 2009 JUNE | | 2008 | | Monthly | Monthly real | YTD | YTD real |
|---|---|---|---|---|---|---|---|---|
| Month: | Monthly | Year to Date | PY Month | PYTD | % change | $$$ change | % change | $$$ change |
| **Revenue** | | | | | | | | |
| Dr. 1 | $ 100,000.00 | $ 600,000.00 | $ 95,000.00 | $ 600,000.00 | 5.3% | $ 5,000.00 | 0.0% | $ - |
| Dr. 2 | $ 120,000.00 | $ 650,000.00 | $ 120,000.00 | $ 600,000.00 | 0.0% | $ - | 8.3% | $ 50,000.00 |
| Dr. 3 | $ 175,000.00 | $ 725,000.00 | $ 225,000.00 | $ 625,000.00 | -22.2% | $ (50,000.00) | 16.0% | $ 100,000.00 |
| *Total:* | *$ 395,000.00* | *$ 1,975,000.00* | *$ 440,000.00* | *$ 1,825,000.00* | *-10.2%* | *$ (45,000.00)* | *8.2%* | *$ 150,000.00* |
| **Expenses** | $ 200,000.00 | $ 950,000.00 | $ 210,000.00 | $ 1,000,000.00 | -4.8% | $ (10,000.00) | -5.0% | $ (50,000.00) |
| Overhead | 50.63% | 48.10% | 47.73% | 54.79% | | | | |
| **New Patients** | | | | | | | | |
| Dr. 1 | 20 | 120 | 18 | 120 | 11.1% | 2 | 0.0% | 0 |
| Dr. 2 | 25 | 130 | 25 | 130 | 0.0% | 0 | 0.0% | 0 |
| Dr. 3 | 30 | 145 | 40 | 130 | -25.0% | (10) | 11.5% | 15 |
| *Total:* | *75* | *395* | *83* | *380* | *-9.6%* | *(8)* | *3.9%* | *15* |
| **Surgeries** | | | | | | | | |
| Dr. 3 | 30.00 | 145.00 | 40.00 | 130.00 | -25.00% | -10 | 11.54% | 15 |
| Practice RVUw | 1750.00 | 15250.00 | 1800.00 | 14200.00 | -2.78% | -50 | 7.39% | 1050 |
| Days in AR | 35.00 | | 45.00 | | -22.22% | | | -10 |

Annotations: $ 50,000.00 — Dr. 3's June drop → Dr. 3's YTD v. PYTD; Good group net gains vs. PYTD

The group looked at the work RVUs for the year using good Dr Hsiao's model to value work in the group, a universal practice management measuring tool, imperfect though it is, to see how they are doing in terms of work. Though Awesome measures this per MD, and keeps the managing partner apprised of significant variation by physician,

**EXHIBIT 26.**

Drs. 1 and 2, P.C.  Practice Snapshot

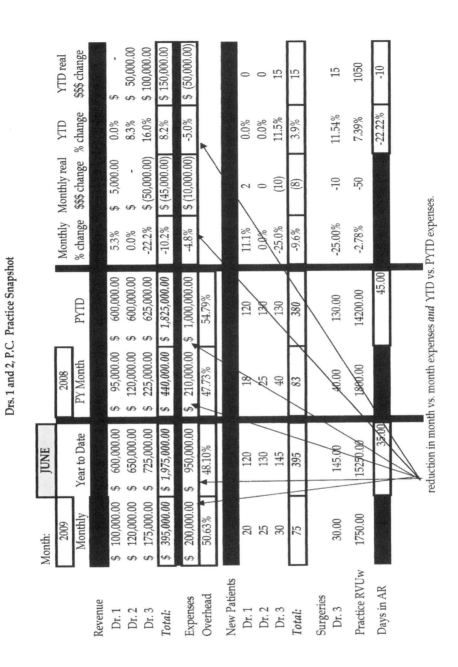

| Month: | 2009 Monthly | Year to Date | 2008 PY Month | PYTD | Monthly % change | Monthly real $$$ change | YTD % change | YTD real $$$ change |
|---|---|---|---|---|---|---|---|---|
| **Revenue** | JUNE | | | | | | | |
| Dr. 1 | $ 100,000.00 | $ 600,000.00 | $ 95,000.00 | $ 600,000.00 | 5.3% | $ 5,000.00 | 0.0% | $ - |
| Dr. 2 | $ 120,000.00 | $ 650,000.00 | $ 120,000.00 | $ 600,000.00 | 0.0% | $ - | 8.3% | $ 50,000.00 |
| Dr. 3 | $ 175,000.00 | $ 725,000.00 | $ 225,000.00 | $ 625,000.00 | -22.2% | $ (50,000.00) | 16.0% | $ 100,000.00 |
| *Total:* | $ 395,000.00 | $ 1,975,000.00 | $ 440,000.00 | $ 1,825,000.00 | -10.2% | $ (45,000.00) | 8.2% | $ 150,000.00 |
| **Expenses** | $ 200,000.00 | $ 950,000.00 | $ 210,000.00 | $ 1,000,000.00 | -4.8% | $ (10,000.00) | -5.0% | $ (50,000.00) |
| Overhead | 50.63% | 48.10% | 47.73% | 54.79% | | | | |
| **New Patients** | | | | | | | | |
| Dr. 1 | 20 | 120 | 18 | 120 | 11.1% | 2 | 0.0% | 0 |
| Dr. 2 | 25 | 130 | 25 | 130 | 0.0% | 0 | 0.0% | 0 |
| Dr. 3 | 30 | 145 | 40 | 130 | -25.0% | (10) | 11.5% | 15 |
| *Total:* | 75 | 395 | 83 | 380 | -9.6% | (8) | 3.9% | 15 |
| **Surgeries** | | | | | | | | |
| Dr. 3 | 30.00 | 145.00 | 40.00 | 130.00 | -25.00% | -10 | 11.54% | 15 |
| Practice RVUw | 1750.00 | 15250.00 | 1800.00 | 14200.00 | -2.78% | -50 | 7.39% | 1050 |
| Days in AR | 35.00 | | 45.00 | | -22.22% | -10 | | |

reduction in month *vs.* month expenses *and* YTD *vs.* PYTD expenses.

they present the data in an aggregated fashion. As you can see, the group has worked 2.78% *less* hard in June than they did last June. This might stand to reason, as we've seen other indicators leading us to this conclusion, such as the drop in practice revenue for the month and the drop in Dr 3's new patient and surgical volumes for the month. So the RVUw drop should not surprise us. We note, too, that there exists a YTD *gain* in RVUws, indicating the group worked harder YTD than they did in the prior year. Again, our other data might lead us to this same conclusion.

## EXHIBIT 27.

Drs. 1 and 2, P.C. Practice Snapshot

Month: JUNE

| | 2009 Monthly | Year to Date | 2008 PY Month | PYTD | Monthly % change | Monthly $$$ change | Monthly real $$$ change | YTD % change | YTD real $$$ change |
|---|---|---|---|---|---|---|---|---|---|
| **Revenue** | | | | | | | | | |
| Dr. 1 | $ 100,000.00 | $ 600,000.00 | $ 95,000.00 | $ 600,000.00 | 5.3% | $ 5,000.00 | $ - | 0.0% | $ - |
| Dr. 2 | $ 120,000.00 | $ 650,000.00 | $ 120,000.00 | $ 600,000.00 | 0.0% | $ - | $ (50,000.00) | 8.3% | $ 50,000.00 |
| Dr. 3 | $ 175,000.00 | $ 725,000.00 | $ 225,000.00 | $ 625,000.00 | -22.2% | $ (50,000.00) | $ (45,000.00) | 16.0% | $ 100,000.00 |
| *Total:* | *$ 395,000.00* | *$ 1,975,000.00* | *$ 440,000.00* | *$ 1,825,000.00* | -10.2% | $ (45,000.00) | | 8.2% | $ 150,000.00 |
| **Expenses** | $ 200,000.00 | $ 950,000.00 | $ 210,000.00 | $ 1,000,000.00 | -4.8% | $ (10,000.00) | | -5.0% | $ (50,000.00) |
| Overhead | 50.63% | 48.10% | 47.73% | 54.79% | | | | | |
| **New Patients** | | | | | | | | | |
| Dr. 1 | 20 | 120 | 18 | 120 | 11.1% | 2 | 0 | 0.0% | 0 |
| Dr. 2 | 25 | 130 | 25 | 130 | 0.0% | 0 | 0 | 0.0% | 0 |
| Dr. 3 | 30 | 145 | 40 | 130 | -25.0% | (10) | | 11.5% | 15 |
| *Total:* | 75 | 395 | 83 | 380 | -9.6% | (8) | | 3.9% | 15 |
| **Surgeries** | | | | | | | | | |
| Dr. 3 | 30.00 | 145.00 | 40.00 | 130.00 | -25.00% | -10 | | 11.54% | 15 |
| Practice RVUw | 1750.00 | 15250.00 | 1800.00 | 14200.00 | -2.78% | -50 | | 7.39% | 1050 |
| Days in AR | | 35.00 | 45.00 | | -22.22% | -10 | | | |

Dr. 3's new patient levels have dropped in June but he's accounted for the lion's share of NP growth YTD vs. PYTD.

Lastly, the group is concerned with its days in AR, a measurement of how quickly the money that is charged out is coming back to the practice in terms of revenue. We note a drop of 10 days in AR, which is nice. That may indicate a couple of things: we're either collecting better, our staff is writing more off (legitimately or not), or we are not charging as much and the money that is out there to be collected is beginning to dry up. Think of it like an oil well that may be running dry. Awesome makes a note to check, and include in next month's numbers, a measurement of charges. With the group working harder, though, they should also be charging more, unless they have lowered the value of their charges, which no group would do. Also, the lowered AR

**EXHIBIT 28.**

Drs. 1 and 2, P.C. Practice Snapshot

| Month: JUNE | 2009 Monthly | 2009 Year to Date | 2008 PY Month | PYTD | Monthly % change | Monthly real $$$ change | YTD % change | YTD real $$$ change |
|---|---|---|---|---|---|---|---|---|
| **Revenue** | | | | | | | | |
| Dr. 1 | $ 100,000.00 | $ 600,000.00 | $ 95,000.00 | $ 600,000.00 | 5.3% | $ 5,000.00 | 0.0% | $ - |
| Dr. 2 | $ 120,000.00 | $ 650,000.00 | $ 120,000.00 | $ 600,000.00 | 0.0% | $ - | 8.3% | $ 50,000.00 |
| Dr. 3 | $ 175,000.00 | $ 725,000.00 | $ 225,000.00 | $ 625,000.00 | -22.2% | $ (50,000.00) | 16.0% | $ 100,000.00 |
| *Total:* | *$ 395,000.00* | *$ 1,975,000.00* | *$ 440,000.00* | *$ 1,825,000.00* | -10.2% | $ (45,000.00) | 8.2% | $ 150,000.00 |
| Expenses | $ 200,000.00 | $ 950,000.00 | $ 210,000.00 | $ 1,000,000.00 | -4.8% | $ (10,000.00) | -5.0% | $ (50,000.00) |
| Overhead | 50.63% | 48.10% | 47.73% | 54.79% | | | | |
| **New Patients** | | | | | | | | |
| Dr. 1 | 20 | 120 | 18 | 120 | 11.1% | 2 | 0.0% | 0 |
| Dr. 2 | 25 | 130 | 25 | 130 | 0.0% | 0 | 0.0% | 0 |
| Dr. 3 | 30 | 145 | 40 | 130 | -25.0% | (10) | 11.5% | 15 |
| *Total:* | *75* | *395* | *83* | *380* | -9.6% | (8) | 3.9% | 15 |
| **Surgeries** | | | | | | | | |
| Dr. 3 | 30.00 | 145.00 | 40.00 | 130.00 | -25.00% | -10 | 11.54% | 15 |
| Practice RVUw | 1750.00 | 15250.00 | 1800.00 | 14200.00 | -2.78% | -50 | 7.39% | 1050 |
| Days in AR | 35.00 | | 45.00 | | -22.22% | | | -10 |

Drop in AR days.

Drop in month RVUs but gain in YTD RVUs.

Dr. 3's month drop in sx volume *but* increase in YTD sx.

may be part of the reason why our revenues have increased. Staff might be collecting better and more aggressively.

What is our summary of this group, year to date vs the prior year to date? Well, the group looks, based on the items it's measuring, pretty darned good. The numbers were down for the month and we've divined that Dr 3 was out of pocket for a week or so. But YTD, the numbers are up nicely and we're controlling our costs. So Awesome the administrator deserves some kudos and Dr 3, we learned, *earned* that vacation!

And now a couple of take aways. One month usually is not fatal, but in my humble opinion, it's worth looking at. The bumps usually smooth out over time, and if they do not, you need to take corrective action. Data is dangerous to use in a vacuum and I've watched MDs massage and move data to fit their needs. If you aggregate enough data, it should lead you down the right path to a sound decision or determination. One component out of context, though, could cause some problems. Always peel back the layers of the onion. The more data, in easy to understand chunks, the better the group will run. But don't "over data." It can confuse and irritate MDs who don't review these numbers on a daily basis and may not understand the data out of context.

## A PARTING SHOT ACROSS THE BOW

You didn't pay all of this money for nothing. I mean, you want to make sure you've received some return on your investment. So tear out these pages, or use the attached Appendices, and begin to aggregate your data. Then winnow that knowledge base down to a few select practices that make your toes wiggle.

Remember, you won't get all of the things you dream about. People seldom do. This would be medical practice nirvana, a state where perfection is out there but most probably not attainable. But the right mix of capable practice staff and management coupled with intimately involved physicians can get you 1 step closer to nirvana.

Ok, I'm no rocket scientist. I've been in health care for 20 years and even I can gain something via osmosis or, as I like to think of it, overexposure or prolonged exposure to health care management. I rather think of it akin to being in the sun for long periods of time. In any event, I know a thing or two about how to run a health care operation. As with any business, the goal is to run an efficient entity and offer a fair return to the shareholders. I'm a firm believer in the theory that good clinicians *deserve*, based on the quality delivery of their care, to earn a good wage. You do not want some underpaid hack snaking a cath tube up your leg. You don't want the guy who finished last in his class (it's a euphemism, so don't be offended if you were last in your class) performing a cataract surgery on you. So, as in the business world, it's reasonable to hope, nay assume, that the guy and gal who were tops get paid tops to be leaders, innovators, creators. These folks should be handsomely rewarded for moving their chosen clinical specialty forward with innovation, drive, and sacrifice. There is nothing shared in this sacrifice unless you've shared it with a spouse.

I said that to say this: the way to generate money in health care (as we discussed) is to see more patients and to do so efficiently. But you need to understand this, completely and fully: this does not mean performing **unnecessary care**. I *firmly* believe that clinicians can make a fair wage by delivering quality care and working efficiently. Remember, there's no money tree out there, so as soon as you disabuse yourself of that notion, you'll be off to a great start. The only way to generate revenue in this odd business model is to offer **great** clinical care and see as many patients as you comfortably can while offering the balance between clinical care and volume. There's no magic bullet; you people are the widget makers, and if you aren't in the office, the widgets aren't getting made and the business isn't generating any revenue. And, though some MDs have tried to posit it, and I *really have heard it*, you **cannot** see fewer patients, work **less**, and make more money, it just ain't economically feasible. Model below:

CPT® code x visits x net charge = revenue

99203 x 5 x $100 = $500

99203 x 3 x $100 = $300

If you can make this model work, copyright the formula and get to selling it.

Given the recent arguments in the country of late, this is **essential** to point out in a sensible, logical, and intellectually viable discussion on the ills of our health care system. The wages a clinician makes correlate, in some manner, with the amount of care given. Whether that's a direct (eat what you treat) or an indirect (you run an efficient group practice with a shared productivity component) correlation, your income will depend on your patient treatment and your efficient use of your resources.

Do I know everything? Of course not. But in this business, if I don't know the answer, I know who to get you to in order to get the right answers. And counter to what the populists in recent media forums would like to portray, we have the best health care system in the world. As with anything of this kind, it is not without its faults and fissures. But it provides the best care available.

My parting words of wisdom for you:

1. Don't overextend yourself financially. You're about to make a pretty fair wage. One thing to avoid is the desire to consume too much. I've seen many physicians dig themselves financial holes when times were good with the practice that later became massive financial craters when times were difficult. Consumption, of course, is fine when balanced.

2. Don't become romantically involved with staff members. I know that seems intuitive, but the impact of an office relationship gone bad can not only have long-lasting effects, it raises the specter of harassment lawsuits, something neither you nor your partners need to endure.

3. Most importantly, love what you do and do what you love. The practice of medicine can still return to physicians a fair living. As I said earlier, don't get greedy and "don't become a partner."

4. Lastly, remember what matters; family, friends, relationships that craft your life and your life experiences. Jobs can come and go and, remember what was stated earlier in the book: "Your job will never love you back." Remember that; your job

will *never* love you back. So make sure you take the time, make the time, to spend with those around you who(m) you hold dear; this venture called life is short and must be embraced in all corners. So go live it!

Good luck and good hunting.

## SUMMARY

I'm proud of you. You made it this far. It's my hope that you enjoyed the book and, if we've accomplished what I'd delineated in the early pages of this manuscript, you've gained a simple and basic understanding into how to look for, and at, a practice to join. We contemplated the inside of the practice, the outside, and how practices function. Those were the key take aways from this endeavor.

This was not meant to offer you insight into $E=MC^2$ or define $\pi$ to a finite point. No, the intent of this book was to offer you an understanding, at least in small part, of the business you're about to enter. If I've done that, I think I've done my job.

I don't expect you to be an expert in practice management nor the day-to-day operations of the practice. I do expect you to come to the table a little better armed, with more of an understanding, and maybe put yourself in a better position to succeed. It's my true feeling that what I've boiled down into these pages can help you to that end; can give you an advantage over your predecessors.

## REFERENCES

1. http://en.wikipedia.org/wiki/Qui_tam
2. *Performance and Practices of Successful Medical Groups*, MGMA
3. CPT 2006: Current Procedural Terminology Standard Edition; AMA
4. Commercial Collection Agency Section of the Commercial Law League of America, http://www2.ccaa collect.com/rate.html
5. Webster's New Collegiate Dictionary, G&C Merriam Co., 1979
6. http://www.nasdaq.com/asp/ExtendFund.asp?&kind=&symbol=unh&symbol=&symbol=&symbol =&symbol=&symbol=&symbol=&symbol=&symbol=&symbol=&selected=unh&FormType= &mkttype=&pathname=&page=full
7. http://www.nasdaq.com/asp/ExtendFund.asp?&kind=&symbol=aet&symbol=&symbol=&symbol =&symbol=&symbol=&symbol=&symbol=&symbol=&symbol=&selected=aet&FormType=&mkt type=&pathname=&page=full
8. http://www.nasdaq.com/asp/ExtendFund.asp?&kind=&symbol=CI&symbol=&symbol=&symbol =&symbol=&symbol=&symbol=&symbol=&symbol=&symbol=&selected=CI&FormType=&mkt type=&pathname=&page=full
9. http://www.aishealth.com/ManagedCare/CompanyIntel/ExecComp.html
10. Medicare Website
11. http://www.cms.hhs.gov/SustainableGRatesConFact/Downloads/sgr2006f.pdf, p.1
12. CBO Economic and Budget Issue Brief, September 6, 2006, p.2; http://www.cbo.gov/ftpdocs/ 75xx/doc7542/09-07-SGR-brief.pdf
13. *ibid*
14. http://www.bcbsphysiciansettlement.com/

## Cuomo: Aetna, CIGNA May Deceive Patients

Bloomberg News
August 17, 2007

Aetna Inc. and CIGNA Corp. may be deceiving patients who rely on the insurers' physician-ranking programs, steering them to cheaper doctors rather than those who are most qualified, New York Attorney General Andrew Cuomo said.

Cuomo's office said in a statement that it asked the companies in letters to justify the programs. Health insurance companies create physician-ranking programs to recommend certain doctors and specialists to patients.

"This program carries significant risk of causing consumer confusion, if not deception," Linda Lacewell, counsel for economic and social justice in the attorney general's office, said in a letter to James E. Brown, Aetna's general counsel. "The attorney general is committed to fostering transparency on behalf of consumers."

Last month, Cuomo asked UnitedHealth Group Inc. not to introduce a doctor-ranking system in New York without his approval. The company planned to introduce such a program in October, he said. He said in today's statement that he and the company are in talks about the program.

Insurers have a profit motive to recommend doctors who charge less, not necessarily those who are most qualified, Cuomo said in today's statement. Patients who choose not to go to the preferred doctors may end up paying more, he said.

"We learned about the letter today and are still in the process of reviewing it, so it would be inappropriate to make any substantive comments," CIGNA spokesman Wendell Potter said in an e-mailed statement. "We take the attorney general's concerns seriously and will respond to his request for information."

"We will cooperate fully," Aetna spokeswoman Cynthia Michener said in an e-mailed response to questions. Aetna created the lists to help patients choose the best doctor based on accepted standards, and doctors can provide information to correct data they think is wrong, Michener said. The first criterion is quality of care, "only then, cost," she said.

"Our program is designed to raise consumer awareness of differences among health care practices that can affect both the effectiveness and cost of care and treatment," UnitedHealth spokesman Tyler Mason said.

**Copyright © 2007, *The Hartford Courant***

## UnitedHealth settles with N.Y. for nearly $4 million

Health Imaging News  |  September 7, 2007  |  Top Stories

As part of a multi-state settlement, UnitedHealthcare, an insurance subsidiary of the Minneapolis-based UnitedHealth Group, will pay New York state $3.7 million following a probe of the insurer's claims processing system, according to *New York Business.com.*

The complete settlement agreement was $13 million and involved 36 states as well as the District of Columbia. The state of N.Y. will receive an additional $320,000 under a separate agreement regarding the insurer's violations of the state's payment statute, claim appeal rules and other regulations.

The Department of Insurance alleged that the investigation of UnitedHealthcare yielded "many errors in claim processing," such as incorrectly applying fees and deductibles, as reported in *New York Business.com.* UnitedHealthcare was also accused of violating prompt payment rules, even after the payor was made aware of its errors.

In accordance with the settlement, delayed UnitedHealthcare claims payments will be reviewed and reprocessed with applicable interest dating back to Jan. 1, 2003. Also, the health insurer has agreed to implement a national improvement plan that will be in effect through the end of 2010, which will subject them to multi-state monitoring of the marketing practices.


## UnitedHealthcare agrees to $12 million settlement with states

By Lydell C. Bridgeford
September 11, 2007
http://ebn.benefitnews.com/asset/article/163508/index.html

UnitedHealthcare has agreed to pay $12 million in fines to 36 states and the District of Columbia regarding multistate investigations into its claims practices.

Some states alleged that the health plan made many errors in claim processing, such as failing to apply fee schedules and deductibles correctly. In addition, state officials criticized the insurer for its handling of claim appeals and consumer complaints, arguing that the company was slow to correct problems, even when notified by state regulators.

In the settlement, UnitedHealthcare neither admitted nor denied the regulatory findings. The settlement requires UnitedHealthcare to investigate, pay or deny claims in a timely fashion. In addition, the company must ensure that claim payments are accurate and that interest is paid when required. The agreement also compels the company, a unit of UnitedHealth Group, to improve its response time to claims-related correspondence.

Patients and health care providers now can provide missing information that is needed for processing before claims close, thus ensuring that claim files contain all necessary documentation.

New York and Florida, which took part in the settlement negotiation, earned the largest payouts—$4 million and $2.7 million, respectively. Arkansas, Connecticut and Iowa also took part in the agreement.

"Consumers and providers deserve timely claims payments, accurate benefit statements and prompt consideration of appeals," says Superintendent Eric Dinallo of the New York Insurance Department. Florida Insurance Commissioner Kevin McCarty comments, "We want to promote a healthy market as regulators, but we also want companies to know we are watching out for our consumers' best interests."

"This new, forward-thinking approach focuses the regulatory process for the states and our company on a practical set of uniform performance standards, while providing clearer and more meaningful means of assessing how well we are serving customers," Kenneth Burdick, CEO of United Healthcare, says.

*Appendix 2*

## CHECKLIST

### Job Search:

***Where in the US do you want to be?***

- East/West/Midwest?
  - Do you want to practice near family or as far away from family as humanly possible?
  - Do you love the coast (left or right)?
  - If you're married, have you and your spouse reached an agreement on geography?

***Urban/suburban:***

- Big city/small suburb?
  - How many physicians are there per 100,000 people?
    - In your specialty, how many physicians are there in the suburb/city of your choice?
  - Basic question: how many MDs are there?

***Lifestyle:***

- Cultural aesthetic of the area
- Night life, theater, fine dining, social happenings, professional sports franchises
- Length of commute/mass transit system
- Places of worship
- School quality

***Payer mix in the area:***

- Dominant payer in the area?

*Helpful note: commercial payers normally reimburse more than Medicare.*

- Check % of mix:
  - BC/BS—          %
  - United—          %
  - Aetna—          %
  - Cigna—          %
  - Medicare—          %
  - Medicaid—          %
  - Self pay—          %
  - Uninsured—          %
  - ***Total:***          ***100%***

*Helpful note: it would be nice if the majority of business was from private pay, especially if the payer reimburses above the Medicare allowable amount.*

▪ Which payer generally dominates your specialty?

*Helpful note: ophthalmology and the retina subspecialty, for instance, might have Medicare as its dominant payer due to the age demographic of the patient base.*

▪ How much revenue might you generate in a good year?

### Malpractice environment:

▪ What is the malpractice history in the area? (eg, case history)

▪ What is the history in your specialty?

▪ Do juries in the area generally side with the physician or the patient?

▪ Does the practice you are interviewing with have any open claims?

▪ What does the practice pay for med/mal coverage per year?

### Physician supply/demand:

More MDs in the area, in your specialty, and in a high-demand area of the country *may* drive down your potential compensation.

### Type of practice:

▪ Hospital-based, academic, private practice

  • Private practice

  — **Solo:**

    ◆ Is there partnership?

    ◆ Have other MDs come before you?

    ◆ If yes, average length of stay with the practice?

    ◆ If an MD has left, what is their current status?

    ◆ Is the solo clinician looking for a partner or employee?

    ◆ Are there reasons the solo MD is still solo?

    ◆ Does the solo MD have a habit of chasing away all potential partners?

    ◆ Does s/he have a history of bringing along new associates only to cut them loose at partnership?

    ◆ Will the solo practitioner allow you to offer input into the practice?

    ◆ Does the practice utilize extenders? (Physician Assistant, Nurse Practitioner, Registered Nurse)

    ◆ Will you have input in solo group or survive as a worker bee? If worker, are you ok with that?

    ◆ What is the practice's quality of life?

    ◆ What is the call schedule?

  — **Group: single or multi-specialty group**

    ◆ Large or small group?

- ° In the area of the country you've settled on, do you *need* to be in a large group for protection?
- ° Single specialty
  - – Eg, ophthalmology with the broad spectrum covering most ophthalmology subspecialties like retina, glaucoma, and cornea
- ° Multi-specialty
  - – Eg, different specialties, sometimes seemingly disparate, under one roof
- ◆ What is the practice's quality of life?
- ◆ What is the call schedule?
- ◆ Does the practice utilize extenders? (Physician Assistant, Nurse Practitioner, Registered Nurse)

***Salary range and negotiations:***
- ▪ Investigate salaries in the area; disparities on high/low end could be telling
- ▪ Research salaries using:
  - • American Medical Association (AMA)
  - • State medical societies
  - • Specialty societies/associations
  - • Practice management associations/societies
    - — Medical Group Management Association (MGMA)
    - — American Medical Group Association (AMGA)
  - • Consultants *strong* in your specialty (so they have knowledge)
- ▪ Negotiation:
  - • Know your position
    - — Demand for physicians in the specialty in the area
    - — The practice's need for physicians
    - — Patient demand (eg, not enough MDs to handle new patient loads)
    - — What revenue might you generate for the practice? This exercise would demonstrate how much value you bring
      - ◆ Exercise: inquire as to how many new patients and rechecks you might see in a year, if fully booked. Plug the numbers in as delineated in this book

*Helpful note: Before hanging your hat on any outside data, make sure it is fairly rigorous and derived from a good sample size.*
  - — Be reasonable in your salary demands (don't overestimate the group's need/desire for you)
  - — Competition in your area of choice might mean you garnering a slightly lower salary
  - — Will they offer a defined list of benefits?
    - ◆ Define the salary

- With what frequency are you paid? Every two weeks (26 x per year)?
- Is there a 401k/profit-sharing plan?
- Vacation/CME time
- CME courses paid? What is the allowance?
- Med/mal covered by group?
  - Do you need to pay any tail (prior acts) coverage if you're changing jobs?
- Is there student loan debt forgiveness?
- Is there a sign-on bonus?
- Is there a car allowance?
- What will call be? What frequency? Do senior physicians get to opt out of call?
- What will the weekly work schedule look like?
  - Daily, how many patients might I see?
    - New patients and consults?
    - Rechecks?

*Helpful note: Try to divine what your tax liability might be when you become a partner.*

### Job search:

Craft a job search log listing:
- Where you've submitted your CV
  - On what date
  - To whom at the practice
  - The status of your submission, and
  - Dates in terms of follow-up

### Other:

Does the practice have other businesses?
- Can you avail yourself of these when you become a partner?
- What is/are the buy-in(s) to those?

### Group:

- What is the physician reporting structure (see organization chart in the book)?
  - Managing partner? His/her name? Time in that role?
  - Board members
  - Executive committee members (if warranted)
  - Administrator? Name and tenure?
- In which office will they put you? Main/satellite?
  - Which MDs work there? Get names and meet them

### Cultural Dynamic:

- What is the group's dynamic?
  - Dynamic of the interview process?

- Names of those MDs involved
- Do all MDs involved provide any input, ask questions?
▪ Practice and MD Vibe
  - Do physicians get along well? (don't need to be best friends, but . . . )
  - Are offices and practice clean and organized?
  - Is equipment new and/or at least maintained?
  - How are employed physicians treated?
    —If larger group, are there methods of dealing with MDs who are outside the line behaviorally?
▪ Median/mean ages of group?
  - Are there older physicians on a retirement track?
  - If there are physicians nearing retirement/work slow-down, is there a defined process?
    —Does the process include call reduction?
    —Does the process include pay reduction?
    —Are these items addressed in partner, employment, operating, or other agreements?
▪ Are there any surprises in the closet?
▪ Does the practice utilize periodic coding audits, either internally or externally?
  - Has the practice been audited due to billing profiles?
  - If audited, how did the practice perform? If coding issues exist, have those been addressed/remedied?
  - Does the practice have a Certified Procedural Coder (CPC)?
▪ What are the work habits of the group?
▪ Is there a penalty committee or overall physician management committee in place?
▪ What is the practice's history with adding new physicians *and* partners?
  - History of bringing on and dumping new associates?
  - How many physicians were hired in last 5 years?
    —How many are still there?
    —How many are partners?
    —Of those who have left, whey did they leave?
      ◆ Can you contact them?
▪ How long is the track to partnership?
  - What does that track involve?
    —Is there a hard asset and/or AR buy-in or simply a par value for stock (eg, 1 share of stock = $10,000)
  - How many physicians have been denied partnership?
    —Of those MDs, how many are still with the group?
  - Explain the buy-in/buy-out?

— What are the details?
- If you elect *not* to be a partner, can you remain employed? (Generally not in your best interest, from a career perspective)
- Are there senior protections written into the senior physicians' contracts? (Eg, a "senior physician" cannot be fired unless other protected physicians feel it is the right move)
- Do the *partners* understand what the structure of the group is?
  - This is also important apropos of your buy-in to the group: do they understand the buy-in and can they elucidate with clarity what it encompasses?

## Business:

### *Strategic Planning:*
- What is the practice's vision?
- What is the practice's mission statement?
- Do they have a strategic plan?
  - If so, can you see it? If you can't see it, how have they measured their goals and have they hit their goals?
  - With what frequency is the plan addressed? Annually?

### *Outside Input:*
- *Accountants:*
  - Does the group have an internal accountant or CFO?
    - If yes, are there outside checks in place?
    - If no, do their outside accountants have health care experience?

How long have they worked for the practice?
- *Attorneys:*
  - Does the practice use attorneys with health care experience?
  - Are their attorneys familiar with:
    - Health Insurance Portability and Accountability Act (HIPAA)
    - Stark laws
    - Fair Market Value (FMV) processes and ramifications
    - Anti-trust/Collusion law
    - Human resources law
- *Other consultants:*
  - Does the practice look for outside assistance on major projects? (Eg, choosing and installing an electronic medical records [EMR] system?)
    - If so, do they have a request for proposal (RFP) process in place to fully vet vendors?
- *Outsourced work:*
  - Does the practice outsource:

    — Staffing?
    — Billing?
    — Collections?
    — Coding?
    — Other?
- If so, have outcomes been quantified and/or measured?
  — If so, have they been successful?

## Management:

- What is the business management structure (vs the partner structure)?
  - Is there a functioning Board or Executive Committee?
  - Is there a managing partner (MP) to work with the administrator?
    — If so, does the MP position have a defined role and service parameter?
    — Is it compensated?
  - Is there an administrator?
    — If so, how long has s/he been with the group?
    — What is his/her background and skill set(s)?
  - What other senior management is there?
    — Is there enough management staff to handle multiple sites if practice has multiple locations?

## Operations:

- What is the practice's overhead ratio?

*Helpful note: many groups run ~50% overhead; generally $0.50 of each dollar goes out to costs, $0.50 gets returned to shareholders. The overhead rate varies based on specialty.*

  - Fixed costs—costs that exist whether or not patients are seen. Eg, facility rent, equipment costs
  - Variable costs—costs that vary based on use
  - Do employed physicians fall above or below the line?
- What are the practice's staffing costs as a percent of revenue? (Should be between 20%–25% of revenues, ideally)
- What are the occupancy expenses? (should be about 6%–8% of revenues)
- What are the equipment costs (percent of revenue dependent upon specialty; eg, family practice might spend less on equipment than private practice cardiology)
- Does the practice have a budget?
  - If yes, is it actively monitored for variances?
  - If not, do they at least review costs with some regularity?
- Days outstanding in accounts receivable (AR)?
  - Gross AR?

- Net AR?

*Helpful note: CHARGES have NOTHING to do with revenue!!! Practices will never receive their entire charged fee, and if they do, their fees need to be reviewed.*

- Are physician and office (if multiple offices) productivity measured?
    - If so, with what metric? RVUs? RVUw? Collections?
    - Are these measures benchmarked against any other data, either inside the group or outside, specialty-specific?
- Does the group have outstanding debt (outside of equipment leases)?
    - If so, for what duration of time?
- Does the group manage their payer contracts?
    - If so, who manages them and what is the process?
    - Have they experienced success negotiating with commercial payers?
        — If so, did they do this internally or employ an external consultant?
    - Does the group know what they get for *each* procedure from *each payer?*
    - Do they, and have they, measured reimbursement as a percentage of the Medicare fee schedule?
    - Does the practice have an active plan in place for appealing and verifying that reimbursements are accurate as per agreed-upon fee schedules?
- Does the group have any technology or other capital initiatives in the works?
    - EMR/EHR?
    - New ultrasound machine?
    - New CT machine?
- Is there a solid practice management system in place?
    - Is the reporting flexible, downloadable, usable in spreadsheet formulas?
    - Are the reports accurate?
    - Is there an IT manager or someone with IT skills to manage the system?
        — If not, is the job farmed out to a qualified individual?
        — Are there ample system protections in place? Security, backup, offsite data storage?

NOTES: